LEAVE WORRIES NOW
BE HAPPY ENJOY LIFE

With the blessing of
GOD GANESHA

LEAVE WORRIES NOW
BE HAPPY ENJOY LIFE

BLESSING OF LORD SHIVA

**LEAVE WORRIES NOW
BE HAPPY ENJOY LIFE**

OMKAR

**LEAVE WORRIES NOW
BE HAPPY ENJOY LIFE**

BLESSINGS OF GOD SHIVA

AND GODESS PARVATI

"OM NAMAH SHIVAY"

LEAVE WORRIES NOW

LEAVE WORRIES NOW
BE HAPPY ENJOY LIFE

ABOUT THE BOOK

Leave Worries Now- Be Happy Enjoy Life, is a very interesting book to read and to lead a happy life. The feeling of happiness or sadness is within us. Yes Worries can surely destroy you. The only way out is to be careful bold and be strong. It is said that worry is purely our own matter. Though it has got something to do with our external circumstances. But there are certainly some positive factors within us that keep us happy and there is something negative within us also which keep us unhappy.

Happy living through positive and good thoughts, is nothing more than that of living a normal life free from undue pressures, problems and tensions. If we want to live a good and happy life then we need to get rid of the negativity within us which makes us unhappy. Negative approach always complicates the problems and increases unhappiness. Most of us do the fatal mistake of looking outwards for happiness rather than looking inwards. Be positive, be strong, be bold and be courageous you are sure to find the feeling of happiness within you.

Even if we are having a bad day, think of some good things that may come our way, either later that day, tomorrow, next week, or next moment. When everything seems to be beyond our control, it's almost too easy for us to slip into the grasp of negativity and unhappiness. To avoid sadness we must strive to abolish this sort of thinking through the power of thinking positively and generate the feeling of happiness within us.

The art of sweet living is not a complicated kind of art difficult to learn rather a simple art of happy living feeling well, eating well, and thinking well.

What we need to do is just to tune up our mind to enjoy every moment of life and let the sweet happiness follow us. This is something that needs to be looked into thoroughly. We need to focus on the positive aspects of lives, rather than on the negative setbacks and enjoy every moment of life happily and merrily. Enjoy your life with cheerful talks. Be happy and cheerful. We must remember that happy living is the reward of sweet and positive thinking. We ought to remember, only the positive thinking can bring happiness in our lives. If we cannot think positively, you cannot live happily. Be our own teacher or adviser we ought to look everything with a positive angle. Let us find something good even in most critical moments of our life and let us make positive thinking the basis of our happy living. It's a matter of thought that fools worry about the circumstances on which they have no control. The wise live on positive good and happy thoughts. A sound and positive happiness is all around. It's not far away from us. If we do not want to live happy, it's up to us. It's our own choice. We must not blame others, nor should we blame our fate or external circumstances. Another thing is that feeling confident affects the way we perceive our situations and how we decide to manage them. Think that by being more optimistic we alter our approaches to situations and take on them in a healthier manner; we think of alternatives and act according to better outcomes. All our efforts lead us to good and happy living. If we think we are positive and happy, it will be positive. It does not say to stick our heads in the soil; rather it says to think positive. Interestingly it does not say feel positive it says think positive and that is the real meaning to remain happy. Positive thinking, good and happy thoughts make us to live happily. Happiness does not come alone, it adds our minds body and soul to remain in constant touch with each other.

We have to remove negative thoughts and create and atmosphere to be happy in our lives. There are many fear factors that are reasoning us to be unhappy and the main reason being that our heart and our feelings which are more susceptible to fear and worry then the mind. We do the worrying in our minds but it is our emotions that make us more worried not our brains. When the heart senses the possibility of loss it can start panicking and then uses the mind to worry and many times tries to manipulate the brain in dealing with the fear. The heart desires something and gets excited about it and then it manipulates the mind to assure that it will get it. Although the brain can control the emotions and knowledge can proceed all. However when it comes to response time the brain is slower than the emotions. That is which explains why we say or do things and then regret them. It would be very hard to tell someone who is worried to feel happy. But if you tell him to think positive that is something even a worried person can do. We need to use our mind to think to be happy and positive. Our objective in life should be to train ourselves to wait for the brain to show up before we say or do anything. Fear usually comes from the emotions and thinking positive is something the brain is capable of doing, making happy living as the key to success. Just think of sweet and happy living. This simple task can be done by thinking positive as it brings positive results in its wake; when you react in a positive way to a negative situation you usually get positive in return and the feeling of happiness is born in you. Positive mental attitude is effective in many ways. There are limits to the effectiveness of positive and happy thinking. Do we try to assume that the persons who are not treating us the way we should be treated are themselves in pain and needs our love and advice to be happy in life and lead a good, sweet and happy life?

It is therefore a must for us to learn and understand r that we need to be positive first and we must think to be happy in the interest of our sweet and happy living.

BALDEV BHATIA

AUTHOR

LEAVE WORRIES NOW
BE HAPPY ENJOY LIFE

PREFACE

An established author, writer and consultant Baldev Bhatia
shares with millions of curious readers the real knowledge
of happiness by letting them know more about themselves
in detail through their in born qualities along with the help
of the positive living qualities possessed by them and to
ward off the negativity in them and also get to know the
ways as how to live happily. The worries adopted by them,
the negative forces influencing them, need to be discarded
for a sweet and happy living. A thought of penning down
the wonders of this interesting and mystic manuscript of
happy and sweet living with the methods to ward off the
negativity influencing the masses has lured the author cum
astrologer to bring to the millions of readers the real
knowledge of sweet and happy living by letting them know
more about themselves in detail with the help of
astrological science. With the guidance of this manuscript
the reader will tend to know more about themselves
through their zodiac signs, their habits, characteristics;
appearances; their personality; profession, career; business,
finances, their match with other zodiac signs; romance,
marriage, weakness their health and disease and finally the
negative forces possessed by them and to ward of this
negativity factor charming them to become more powerful
so that they can lead a sweet, good and happy life. This
Microscopy of Good and Happy Living is based on the
practical experience of the author who has meet several
thousand people having negativity in their personal lives
and those leading a miserable life totally being depressed
and dejected who have bitterly failed to lead a good and
happy life.

The main purpose of writing this manuscript is to impart the basic knowledge of how to become bold, strong, courageous, and how to throw away the negativity in them. This manuscript reveals a whole lot of information when one is in search for the truth of happy living. The author also shares his experience with his readers through his published books "Microscopy of Astrology", Microscopy of Numerology", Microscopy of Remedies, Microscopy of

Transiting Planets five volumes and also guides his readers to achieve their personal goals with ease and assist them to overcome all the problems, crises, and the unforeseen negatives forces, in their lives by parting with depression, dejection disappointment and by adopting the beautiful ways of enjoying a sweet good and happy living.

This book goes to reveal, ascertaining the real facts of life and the destiny as to what is stored for each and every reader in his or her future. Various chapters have been covered and maximum emphasis have been paid to cover the subjects pertaining to the significance of happiness by reading different charts; different zodiac signs, planets and their placements in different houses and signs; affliction of planets with the interpretation of the major period and the meaning of the birth sign.

Author and Astrologer Baldev Bhatia have put his entire life experience in promoting positivity and happiness among his clients through this mystic science of Astrology. He has done so in order to serve millions of curious readers with a good intension of imparting them the basic knowledge of how to become a happy person in life.

The author-cum astrologer has been associated with general public for the past forty five years and has been practicing phycology and pubic healing.

His intension is also to guide the readers to achieve their personal goals with ease and would assist them to overcome all the problems, crises, speed breakers and the unforeseen negatives forces, in their lives and always to ward of the dejection negativity in their lives and to lead a happy life. The Author's main object and message, through this manuscript to his readers is to spread, peace, love happiness to the entire world and tries to guide his readers to ward off unhappiness sadness and hatred among them. He has done his best to reveal to his readers to attain positivity in way or manner irrespective of all the hardships and to attain a path of glory by getting away from their weakness of negative thinking and discarding forever the negative attitude, to be bold to be strong and e courageous, through which they can lead a sweet good happy and prosperous life. This book also intends to guide the readers to achieve their personal goals with ease that would assist them to overcome all the problems, difficulties crises, in their lives, as not to get worried or disheartened if the influence of the transiting planets is weak, guesting depressing, unfavorable and disappointing.

This books goes to emphasis as how to lead a sweet good and happy life eve if the influence of the MahaDasha is good, it brings good or positive changes or events in life. But if the influence is unfavorable it gives undesired results.

One needs to understand that no matter what aspect a transiting planet makes to an individual he needs to hold on his nerves to be bold to be strong and to be positive in life whatever be the circumstances governing his future and the positive energy that is already stored in him. The chapters in the book are very useful, purposeful, and a pin point to the service of mankind. He wishes success for all his readers.

The author would definitely like to express his sincere
thanks to Ms. Alpa Shah Director, Travel Company of UK,
for helping and encouraging him to pen down this book in
the interest of depressed and dejected and the so called
unhappy persons of this universe. The author is also
grateful and thankful to for publishing this
Book.

BALDEV BHATIA
AUTHOR

LEAVE WORRIES NOW
BE HAPPY ENJOY LIFE

ABOUT THE AUTHOR

Astrology has stood the test of times ever since it revealed the mystery and the mastery of the ancient wisdom of forecasting the influence of the stars on human bodies. The author Baldev Bhatia a renowned and world famous astrologer has penned several simple books on astrology- this mysterious subject that reveals the true perception of knowing oneself through the art of prediction. Professionally the author has put his entire life experience in promoting Astrology in various fields with a view to serve the millions of curious readers of this mystic science and with the intension of imparting them the real knowledge of astrology through various marvelous scriptures. The Astrologer has been associated with astrology for the past forty five years and has been practicing astrology in various forms. The Author-cum Astrologer has been in touch with general public and has been practicing phycology and pubic healing. His intension is to guide his readers to achieve their personal goals with ease that would assist them to overcome all the problems, crises, speed breakers and the unforeseen negatives forces, in their lives so as not to get disheartened or depressed in their lives and finally lead a happy life and peaceful and a sweet life. The author also shares with millions of curious readers the 'real knowledge' by letting them know more about themselves in detail and also about their in born positive qualities, possessed by them and guides them to ward off the negativity in them, by getting to know as how to lead an happy and powerful life.. without caring for the worries troubling them, the negative forces influencing them, which needs to be discarded forever, for a sweet and happy living if the influence of the transiting planets.

The main object of writing this manuscript is to impart the basic knowledge of how to become positive, bold, strong, courageous, and how to throw away the negative forces and become a happy person in life. The author also shares the valuable experience of his life with his readers through this valuable and helpful book.

His published books "Microscopy of Astrology", Microscopy of Numerology", Microscopy of Remedies, Microscopy of Happy Living Microscopy of Positive Living and Microscopy of Positive Thinking also guide his readers to achieve their personal goals with ease and assists them to overcome all the problems, in their lives gracefully which guides them to lead a happy sweet and prosperous life.

His readers have gained good experience going through his useful and purposeful books. His books have made his readers to feel secure, sound and have also encouraged them to face their destiny with immense strength and have also given them the power to face the challenges of this universe with utter confidence zeal and power and are leading a happy life. The author Baldev Bhatia leads way to happiness, success, positivity and advices his people suffering from depression and negativity in their personal lives to wake up and lead a positive and to be happy. After meeting hundreds and hundreds of depressed dejected disappointed and unhappy people from all over the world and people from all walks of life and he being a highly experienced astrologer and consultant in astrology and numerology felt it necessary to write books on Happiness, Love, and on the art of sweet living. His books have also revealed to his readers to attain happiness in their lives so that they could easily achieve their path of glory and also be a brave strong and courageous human being. His books have given gracefully accepted by the people worldwide.

His books have helped the masses to achieve and lead a life full of positivity, boldness, courage happiness and have generated confidence in depressed and dejected people. His books have helped his clients and readers to lead a good, a sweet and happy life. His books have been very different as they guide and help the readers to strengthen their will power and confidence which the readers have lost in today's world. In order to encourage his readers and to help them, in all walks of life the esteem author decided to manuscript the following books in the interest and happiness of the universal world.

1. Microscopy of Astrology

2. Microscopy of Numerology

3. Microscopy of Remedies

4. Microscopy of Happy Living

5. Microscopy of Transiting Planets Vol 1, 2, 3, 4, and 5

6. Microscopy of Positive Living- An Art of Happy Living

7. Microscopy of Positive Thinking – An Art of Good Living

He wishes his readers all the success happiness and prosperity.

He praises God and prays Him with the following words.

"May the Heavens Shower Peace Prosperity and Happiness to All"

"GOD BLESS YOU" "THANKS FOR READING "

BALDEV BHATIA   AUTHOR

DATED 15TH DEC; 2016

LEAVE WORRIES NOW
BE HAPPY ENJOY LIFE

TABLE OF CONTENT

CHAPTER 1

LEAVE WORRIES NOW
BE HAPPY ENJOY LIFE

WHAT IS WORRY?

Thought which are provoking our mind, about the
uncertainties and the negativities, as to what will happen
tomorrow. Worries are repetitive thoughts associated with
feelings of anxiety in anticipation of some negative future
event. Whether the worries are about financial crisis, family
problems, work, health or any topic of concern, the anxious
feelings produced and sustained by the imaginary thoughts
which always distinctly appear to be unpleasant. Worrying
will carry tomorrow's load with today's strength. Worry
will not empty tomorrow of its sorrows, it empties today of
its power and strength. Worries make you to move into
tomorrow ahead of time. Half the worry in the world is
caused by people trying to make decisions before they have
sufficient knowledge on which to base a decision. Why
worry about the future. Just imagine as to what if we just
acted like everything was easy and there was nothing very
serious about it to come in future. Worry often gives a
small thing a big shadow and its surrounding do frightened
with more scary things. Why worry about tomorrow;
concentrate on today happening as for tomorrow will worry
about itself. Each day has its own worries and troubles. If
there is not any solution to the some problem then do not
waste time worrying about it. And if there is a solution to
the problem then why waste time worrying about it. Worry
will never rob tomorrow of its sorrows, but will only deny
today of its meaning happiness and joys.

Worrying is actually a form of superstition and creates false images in our mind and that is the main reason and cause which makes and leads us to this point of imagination. A human being can survive almost anything, as long as he or she sees the end in sight. If something bad or good is to happen it is sure to happen, whether we worry or not. Let us put our energy into today and stop worrying about the future and past. We should not foresee trouble, or worry about what may never happen as past is dead and gone forever and future is uncertain and yet to come. The basic facts we should know about worry. The basic techniques to analyze worry and how to break the worry habit before it breaks us. These are the simple ways where we can concentrate and get rid of worries prevailing in our thoughts. Annalise worry to see and get the reasons and facts of worry. To avoid reoccurrence of worries, concentrate on prayers as prayers are the best source of remedies of the prevailing worries. The more you pray, the less you'll panic. The more you worship, the less you worry. There is nothing that wastes the body like worry, and anyone who has any faith in God should need not to worry about anything whatsoever is to happen in future. We ought to know the basic fundamental of analyzing worries. Worries create unnecessary thoughts and these are caused by people going in for unwanted decisions, fore hand not even knowing as to when a good decision is made and not even having sufficient knowledge about it. We must first study and after carefully weighing all the facts than only come to a powerful decision. Simply making castles in the air won't solve our problems but add more to our vows. Anxiety and worry can go hand in hand.

When anxiety grabs the mind, it is self-perpetuating. Your mind gets clogged with numerous with buts and ifs. Do not worry about your life. Worries are repetitive thoughts associated with feelings of anxiety in anticipation of some negative future event. Yet anxious feelings and the worries that lead to them can prove helpful. It becomes a difficult problem if you are constantly anxious as it will become a hindrance to your everyday life, rather than motivate you to some good and better things. Never worry alone. Worrisome thoughts reproduce faster so one of the most powerful ways to stop the spiral of worry is simply to disclose the worry to a friend. What you will eat or drink; or about your body, what you will wear. If you know that the circumstance is beyond your control or power change than revise it to your liking. Just try to put a stop-less order on your worries. Don't permit little things which become insects of life to ruin your happiness. Co-operate with the inevitable. Decide just how much anxiety a thing may be worth and refuse to give in anymore. All the happiness is not given in one go it comes slowly and slowly.

If your worries center on, an important relationship in your life, pay special attention to remain positive and be happy. To keep yourself happy, treat your worried thoughts as valuable signals. How to keep from worrying about criticism? Simply unjust criticism is often a disguised compliment. It often means that you have aroused jealousy and envy. Let's keep a record of the fool things we have done and criticize ourselves. The utmost cause of worry is your state of depression. Worries are there to motivate information-gathering and problem-solving. Depression is the inability to construct a future.

Depression is inertia. That's the thing about depression: But depression is so insidious, and it compounds daily, that it's impossible to ever see the end. Depressed people think they know themselves, but maybe they only know depression. There are no hopeless than this to get depressed. Our attitude towards suffering and depression becomes very important because it can affect how we cope with suffering when it arises. Depression is nourished by a lifetime of un grieved and unforgiven causes. Never worry about your heart till it stops beating. How can you deal with anxiety? You might try what when you did. A person worried so much that he decided to hire someone to do his worrying for him. Times will change for the better when you change. Worry is a misuse of the imagination. Worry is most often a prideful way of thinking that you have more control over life and its circumstances than you actually do. To keep yourself happy, treat your worried thoughts as valuable signals. These are the fundamental facts you should be familiar about worries. A huge factor to stay happy is to cater your worries around, an important relationship in your life and pay special attention sustaining positive relationships. Worries are there to motivate information gathering and problem-solving. Make your mind firm and do come to a positive decision as come what we will not allow the worries to entire our mind and soul. Once a decision is carefully reached we should get busy carrying out our decisions and should not bother about all the anxieties that are about to come. When we, or any of our colleagues or associates, are about to worry about a problem, we must write it out and think of the following questions:

Instead of worrying about what people say of you, why not spend time trying to accomplish something they will admire. What if we just acted like everything was easy? How would your life be different if you stopped worrying about things we can't control and started focusing on the things we can? Let today be the day. You free yourself from fruitless worry, seize the day and take effective action on things you can change...

LEAVE WORRIES NOW
BE HAPPY ENJOY LIFE

CHAPTER 2

WHAT DO YOU GET OUT OF WORRYING?

You may feel largely uncomfortable, when worries attack your thoughts and mind which makes worrying about a situation an easier option to get depressed and diffused. While you are consuming more worries you are far too busy to do anything else to fix the real problem and would rather find it hard to get into a smart solution. Thus resulting in a fact that you spend your evenings worrying only without even bothering to find some time to search a new job. You get nothing out of worrying except only to think and cry. Another cause of getting worried is the attachment with which your inner soul gets attracted to. Attachment brings worry. If you have a problem and you come up with the answer, you stop worrying immediately. Our minds can be dishonest, persuading us that we are worrying about something, when our deepest fear is entirely different. No-one likes to admit that they've chosen to worry. The first step is to write down your worries, which will help you make sense of them, and then decide on one small step you can take towards a solution. But to be very true no man in this world is free of obstacles or difficulties. Don't make worry your habit. Break this habit and stop all the negative and panic thoughts provoking your mind all the time. If you can't change the past, but you must not ruin the present by worrying about the future.

Joy is what happens to us when we allow ourselves to recognize how good things really are. When we feel worried and depressed, we need to consciously form a smile on our faces and act upbeat until the happy feeling becomes genuine reality. Feelings of depression and hopelessness and or anger are even tougher to cope with on a consistent basis. When you are worried, you not only hurt yourself, but the limited support systems that are still holding on your mind but making you to get more and more worried and nothing is achieved in terms of success except the re-carnation of worries and worries......

Your actions breed confidence and courage. If you want to conquer fear, anger and worry do not sit ideal and just think about it. Let our deep worrying become advance thinking and planning. If you look into your own mind and heart, and you find nothing wrong there, what is there to worry about? Practically nothing what is there to fear about and again nothing? So why worry unnecessarily and make your present and future dark.

LEAVE WORRIES NOW
BE HAPPY ENJOY LIFE

CHAPTER 3

WHY WORRY SO MUCH

Negative thought which are provoking our mind, about the uncertainties and the negativities, as to what will happen tomorrow creates unnecessary worries and worries are repetitive thoughts associated with feelings of anxiety in anticipation of some negative future event which may end in a failure. Whether the worries are about financial crisis, family problems, work, health or any topic of concern, the anxious feelings and negative thoughts produced are always distinctly unpleasant. Annalise positive thinking and stop worry over petty matters. Worrying will carry tomorrow's load with today's strength. Worry will not empty tomorrow of its sorrows, but it tends to empty today of its power and strength. Worries make you to move into tomorrow ahead of time. Half the worry in the world is caused by people trying to make decisions before they have sufficient knowledge on which to base a decision. Their negative thoughts pressurize them to be away from the positivity in their lives as they fail and do not analysis on positive

Generate Positive Thinking

Why worry about the future. Just imagine as to what if we just acted like everything was easy and there was nothing very serious about it to come in future. Worry often gives a small thing a big shadow and its surrounding do frightened with more scary things. Why worry about tomorrow; concentrate on today happening as for tomorrow will worry about itself. Each day has its own worries and troubles. Always think positive.

If there is not any solution to the some problem then do not waste time worrying about it. And if there is a solution to the problem then why waste time worrying about it. Act fast be positive generate positive thinking worries will automatically vanish in the air. But if you tend to worry they will never rob tomorrow of its sorrows, but will only deny today of its meaning happiness and joys. Negative thoughts only produce worries and worrying is actually a form of superstition and creates false images in our mind and that is the main reason and cause which makes and leads us to this point of imagination. A human being can survive almost anything, as long as he or she sees the end in sight and starts analyzing his positive thoughts. We must not forgot that if something bad or good is to happen it is sure to happen, whether we worry or not. Let us put our energy into today and stop worrying about the future and past. We should not foresee trouble, or worry about what may never happen as past is dead and gone forever and future is uncertain and yet to come. Positive Thinking will ward off everything and bring happiness in our lives. The basic facts we should know about worry. The basic techniques to analyze worry and how to break the worry habit before it breaks us. These are the simple ways where we can concentrate and get rid of worries prevailing in our thoughts.

Think Positive and Pray- Why Worry?

Annalise positive thinking by annualizing worry you get to see and get the reasons and facts of worry. To avoid reoccurrence of worries, concentrate on prayers as prayers are the best source of remedies of the prevailing worries. Think Positive and Pray. The more you pray, the less you'll panic. The more you worship, the less you worry. There is nothing that wastes the body like worry, and anyone who has any faith in God should need not to worry about anything whatsoever is to happen in future.

Positive thinking is the creation of good imagination. We must first study and after carefully weighing all the facts than only come to a powerful decision. Simply making castles in the air won't solve our problems but add more to our vows. Anxiety and worry can go hand in hand. When anxiety grabs the mind, it is self-perpetuating. Your mind gets clogged with numerous with buts and ifs. Do not worry about your life. Worries are repetitive thoughts associated with feelings of anxiety in anticipation of some negative future event. Yet anxious feelings and the worries that lead to them can prove helpful. It becomes a difficult problem if you are constantly anxious to know as to the happening of the future. It will become a hindrance to your everyday life, rather than motivate you to some good and better things. Worrisome thoughts reproduce faster so one of the most powerful ways to stop the spiral of worry is simply to disclose the worry to a friend. What you eat or drink; or about your body, what you will wear will add to negativity may discard positive thinking.

Happiness comes with Positive Thinking.

If you know that the circumstance is beyond your control or power change than revise it to your liking. Just try to put a stop-less order on your worries. Don't permit little things which become insects of life to ruin your happiness. Co-operate with the inevitable. Decide just how much anxiety a thing may be worth and refuse to give in anymore. All the happiness is not given in one go it comes slowly and slowly with positive thinking. Have worry under your control. If your worries center around, pay special attention to remain positive and be happy. Keep yourself happy, treat your worried thoughts as valuable signals. How to keep from worrying about criticism? Simply unjust criticism and think positively and do often discard a bad compliment. It often means that you have aroused jealousy and envy.

Let's keep a record of the fool things we have done and
stop criticizing ourselves.

Cause of Worry is Negative Thinking- Think Positive

The utmost cause of worry is our negative thinking as it
leads us to the state of depression. Worries are there to
motivate us and not a mere source of information-gathering
and problems. Dejection and Depression is the inability to
construct a future. Depression is inertia. That's the thing
about depression: But depression is so insidious, and it
compounds daily, that it's impossible to ever see the end.
Depressed people think they know themselves, but maybe
they only know depression. There are no hopeless than this
to get depressed. They never even attempt to think positive.

Times will change for the better-Think Positive

Our negative thinking and attitude towards suffering and
depression becomes very important because it can affect
how we cope with suffering when it arises. Depression is
nourished by a lifetime of un-grieved and unforgiven
causes. Never worry about your heart till it stops beating.
How can you deal with anxiety? You might try what when
you did. A person worried so much that he decided to hire
someone to do his worrying for him. Times will change for
the better when you change. Worry is a misuse of the
imagination. Worry is most often a prideful way of thinking
that you have more control over life and its circumstances
than you actually do. Positive Thinking leads your way to
good and happiness. An art of Good and Happy Living.
Neglect worries keep yourself happy, treat your worried
thoughts as valuable signals. These are the fundamental
facts you should be familiar about worries. A huge factor to
stay happy is to cater your worries around, an important
relationship in your life and pay special attention sustaining
positive relationships. Worries are there to motivate
information gathering and problem-solving.

Make your mind firm and do come to a positive decision as come what we will not allow the worries to entire our mind and soul. Once a decision is carefully reached we should get busy carrying out our decisions and should not bother about all the anxieties that are about to come. When we, or any of our colleagues or associates, are about to worry about a problem, we must write it out and think positively of the questions: Instead of worrying about what people say of you, why not spend time trying to accomplish something they will admire. What if we just acted like everything was easy? How would your life be different if you stopped worrying about things we can't control and started focusing on the things we can? Let today be the day. You free yourself from fruitless worry, seize the day and take effective action on things you can change. We would change ourselves for the betterment if we start thinking in positive terms. Positive thinking is what is required of us and simply worrying about the future things or as to what will happen in the next moment will certainly deprive us of good and happy living that we are about gather or get in the next hour.

LEAVE WORRIES NOW
BE HAPPY ENJOY LIFE
CHAPTER 4

STOP WORRYING?

You may feel largely uncomfortable, when worries attack your thoughts and mind which makes worrying about a situation an easier option to get depressed and diffused. While you are consuming more worries you are far too busy to do anything else to fix the real problem and would rather find it hard to get into a smart solution. Thus resulting in a fact that you spend your evenings worrying only without even bothering to find some time to search a new job. You get nothing out of worrying except only to think and cry. Another cause of getting worried is the attachment with which your inner soul gets attracted to. Attachment brings worry. If you have a problem and you come up with the answer, you stop worrying immediately. Our minds can be dishonest, persuading us that we are worrying about something, when our deepest fear is entirely different. No-one likes to admit that they've chosen to worry. The first step is to write down your worries, which will help you make sense of them, and then decide on one small step you can take towards a solution. But to be very true no man in this world is free of obstacles or difficulties. Don't make worry your habit. Break this habit and stop all the negative and panic thoughts provoking your mind all the time. If you can't change the past, but you must not ruin the present by worrying about the future.

Joy is what happens to us when we allow ourselves to recognize how good things really are. When we feel worried and depressed, we need to consciously form a smile on our faces and act upbeat until the happy feeling becomes genuine reality. Feelings of depression and hopelessness and or anger are even tougher to cope with on a consistent basis. When you are worried, you not only hurt yourself, but the limited support systems that are still holding on your mind but making you to get more and more worried and nothing is achieved in terms of success except the re-carnation of worries and worries Your actions breed confidence and courage. If you want to conquer fear, anger and worry do not sit ideal and just think about it. Let our deep worrying become advance thinking and planning.

LEAVE WORRIES NOW
BE HAPPY ENJOY LIFE

CHAPTER 5

FORGET WORRIES

You may feel largely uncomfortable, when worries attack your thoughts and mind which makes worrying about a situation an easier option to get depressed and diffused. While you are consuming more worries you are far too busy to do anything else to fix the real problem and would rather find it hard to get into a smart solution. Thus resulting in a fact that you spend your evenings worrying only without even bothering to find some time to search a new job. You get nothing out of worrying except only to think and cry. Another cause of getting worried is the attachment with which your inner soul gets attracted to. Attachment brings worry. If you have a problem and you come up with the answer, you stop worrying immediately. Our minds can be dishonest, persuading us that we are worrying about something, when our deepest fear is entirely different. No-one likes to admit that they've chosen to worry. The first step is to write down your worries, which will help you make sense of them, and then decide on one small step you can take towards a solution. But to be very true no man in this world is free of obstacles or difficulties. Don't make worry your habit. Break this habit and stop all the negative and panic thoughts provoking your mind all the time. If you can't change the past, but you must not ruin the present by worrying about the future.

Joy is what happens to us when we allow ourselves to recognize how good things really are. When we feel worried and depressed, we need to consciously form a smile on our faces and act upbeat until the happy feeling becomes genuine reality. Feelings of depression and hopelessness and or anger are even tougher to cope with on a consistent basis. When you are worried, you not only hurt yourself, but the limited support systems that are still holding on your mind but making you to get more and more worried and nothing is achieved in terms of success except the re-carnation of worries and worries. Your actions breed confidence and courage. If you want to conquer fear, anger and worry do not sit ideal and just think about it. Let our deep worrying become advance thinking and planning. If you look into your own mind and heart, and you find nothing wrong there, what is there to worry about? Practically nothing what is there to fear about and again nothing? So why worry unnecessarily and make your present and future dark. All your thoughts, good and bad, are the creation which tends to lead you to a materialistic life and go in to generate unnecessary worries. That is why you must learn to be more positive. The environment and all the experiences in your life are the results of your habitual and dominant thoughts. Negative thoughts could tell us about something that needs special attention when they lead us to the path of worries. We must discover what needs to be done, and think positively to take care of it. Many of us fail to see a negative occurrence and do not think of a replacement of negative thought with positive one. They even do not look for a bright side in every situation.

If we do this for a longer period of time, we become habitual, and it will make a tremendous delay in improving our positive thinking skills. We must remember, everything can be framed positively if we make a restless effort to do so. There are both positive and negative aspects to most situations. We get to choose which ones we will focus on. We can try to catch ourselves when we're being negative and do not try thinking the opposite. There's no sense in worrying about the negatives if these negatives cannot be changed. If we waste energy and happiness on the things we can't change, we'll only make ourselves more frustrated and come to the stage of depression. Negativity is a habit and we often don't realize we're doing ourselves down. Under each negative thought you've written, see if you can spot an alternative way of looking at it, that isn't so negative. There's a world of difference between expecting failure or rejection - so as not to be disappointed when it occurs - and recognizing it as a possibility. It's sensible to look at a situation from all angles and to have a back-up plan to fall back on if need be. People who do this will often see failure as another step on the road to eventual success; but by expecting and envisioning success, there's less likely to be a failure. Let us find some ways of removing negative thoughts and discouraging our worries to be born.

1.   By way of giving a good Smile

The first easiest way is smiling. Many theories have revealed that even a forced smile can lift one's mood. We may also share positivity with others by flashing them with a brilliant smile. Smiling is a reward, not a risk.

The only thing we risk when smiling is a giving ourselves a little more happiness.

2.   By way of having the company of good friends. Keep yourself busy and surround yourself with good friends. Appreciate the people in your life who have stood by you through thick and thin. Count their support which has helped you become more positive, and in the process you will probably help them too.

Good friends help each other in the days of crises and through both the good and bad times. Feel positive about them and feel lucky to have them in your company.

3.   Focus your thoughts on positive imagination Focus your imagination and make efforts on becoming that new positive person. It is much easier to bring about change if you just put your mind to it and change your thoughts into a much more positive direction. We know that it is difficult for us to control things that happen in our lives, but we can, with some effort, control what we think or do in our lives. Positive thinking will make our imagination livelier and we would be able to lead our lives without many worries. Depression, however, has consequences that could ruin your self-esteem, health, and well-being.

LEAVE WORRIES NOW
BE HAPPY ENJOY LIFE

CHAPTER 6

DON'T WORRY -START LIVING

At time we may think that there is no road is left for us from where we can achieve the happiness of our lives. We may also feel that life has become terrible for us to live and we are carrying new hope that someone would come to rescue us. There may be chances that someone who was there with us before might have held on to us when we were on the dark side of the life.

It is important for us to stay open to laughter and humor.

Even when we are facing challenges, it is important for us to stay open to laughter and humor. Sometimes, simply recognizing the potential humor in a situation can lessen our stress and brighten our outlook. Seeking out sources of humor such as watching a funny sitcom or reading jokes online can help us to think more positively.

The experience has taught us that we should buy some strength, hope and positive ness from our loved ones to help ourselves in such a situation rather than surrendering as life is a precious gift of God and is equipped with full of joy and happiness if we help ourselves in these critical moments and live with considerable optimism. Happiness in life comes through the doors of positive thoughts; we do not even realize which one is left open.

We have so many reasons to cry and at the same time plenty of reasons to smile as well.

Keeping our dreams and hope alive might be a reason that success and happiness will come our way again.

We ought to know that happiness alone does not stand for anything, but it is on our way of thinking that how do we keep ourselves happy in life. Ending up our lives does not lead us to our destination but of course proves we are supposed to be cowards who know not to unfold the doors of belief in God and in ourselves. But if our faith is strong enough we will not be let down, rather we would break the knees of sorrows and force it to die and lead happy lives.

We must find out ways to come out of our worries, anxieties and difficulties.

We should not surrender but must find out ways to come out of our worries, anxieties and difficulties. We ought not to indulge ourselves into the darkness of the room but find out the doors to free ourselves from unnecessary fear and worries. We must belief in ourselves and our hearts, and believe in the ones who love us and not the ones whom we love. We must not fall on the negative side of a thing. It is the real time when we keep on revealing the truth of our lives and relations. We should always try to be happy and should think that whatever is happening, it is the positive side. We should accept the situation and fight it with more determination. We must find out ways to come out of our worries, anxieties and difficulties in order for us to lead a happy sweet and good life.

Negative thoughts are our greatest enemies.

We ought to know that advice from people around us will help us to overcome from the any drastic situation. Also we have to always minimize the stress as it gives nothing but takes away joy and happiness from our lives. And finally we need to take things casually and fight with it seriously. A clear minded person looks for good qualities in the other person, whereas a negative mind always looks for the fault in the other person, whereas a negative mind always looks for the fault. An optimist goes forward keeping in mind the past, a pessimist thinks of the future and reverts back to the past.

In fact negative thoughts are our greatest enemies. Experience the happiness in all circumstances by maintaining better relationships.

We need to analyise the reason for our unhappiness.

Whenever we are unhappy, if we analyze the reason for our unhappiness, it is because life is not matching our desires and expectations. We need to know and realize that nobody is perfect or flawless. If we try to change the way we look, talk and behave just to please others, and show our pride we will gradually become such a person that we ourselves won't recognize each other and would start and create unnecessary worries within us and our surrounding without being positive and will not start to live happily. We ought to stop worrying over unnecessary things be positive and live without fear. Living happily is the master key to all problems and worries. Forgot worries discard all problems take them lightly and behave as nothing serious has happened. This way we are sure to overcome all problems and lead a happy life. We need to understand that what people think of us is their concern, and not ours. If they think about us to be, too reticent or proud, it's really not our business. If every time we happen to meet some new fellows, we may wonder and imagine as what they think of us, and with this feeling in us we will never be able to live a trouble-free and hassle free life. We are bound to fall into the trap of unnecessary worries denying us the startup of new and the happy living life.

Positive attitude is a quality of happy living.

We must think rationally. Is it in our hands or can we control what others think about us? Simply we need to ignore them, if we cannot, and live our lives the way we want to and find the ways to leave worries aside and start living a happy life. Let us make our way to happy living. It is a well-known fact that attitude decides how a natives or persons copes up with the day to day events of life.

Attitude is the main influence a person's reaction to a situation in life. It sets the emotional undertone for a person to his likes or dislikes a situation even before he is acquainted with it. Positive attitude is a quality of happy living which is second to none in a human being. We acknowledge our children to say a big thank you from the time to time irrespective they being very little, we teach them to be grateful for everything that they receive. We attach so much importance to this attitude of gratitude that when our children fail to thank someone, we insist that they do it. That is what is needed to be avoided from time to time. We expect this in return from others when we help them or give them a gift. We call a person discourteous and rude when they do not say thank us in return. Though we attach so much importance to this attitude, as we grow into teenage and adult years we find ourselves becoming ungrateful or taking things for granted. We lose touch with the very same qualities that we instill in our children. We take for granted our life, our health, our families, the people in our lives, the things that our loved ones do for us to make our lives easier and things that we possess.

The attitude of positive or happy living speaks a lot about a person.

It denotes about changing negative attitudes and making positive thinking a positive a good habit. Thinking positively and a positive attitude help us to appreciate and value ourselves, our potential and all that we have. It ensures that we do not take our abilities for granted. It makes us look at ourselves as special people with a special set of abilities and potential. It banishes the feelings of inadequacy and insecurity that arises from unfair comparisons with others. It helps us to appreciate people for who they are and not magnify what they are not and their little flaws. It drives away prejudice and makes us approach life with an open mind. It predisposes us to react to the daily events of life in a positive manner and help us to look at the brighter side of life. Make us optimistic.

It gives hope and helps us look forward to life with anticipation making our lives happier and happier day be day. We need to know that positive thinking takes the focus away from what we don't have, to appreciating and making good use of what we have. It is closely connected to our emotional wellbeing and happiness. We feel loved and at peace with ourselves for a major part of our lives when we make this attitude ours. This adds and helps us to get rid of greed, amenity, bitterness, jealousy, and promotes a healthy and nurturing attitude towards others, which in turn gets reciprocated and we feel the sense of healthy living. On the face of it we ought to know that a positive and good living is an attitude that makes you feel good about who you are, what you do, and what your potentials are. This attitude impels you to utilize all that you are endowed with as a person, to achieve the highest possible goals. When we have this attitude, we are able to work without any external pressure to perform but there is sufficient pressure and motivation from within.

Positive thinking and a positive attitude of happy life is a joy for ever

The possessing of happy living is like any other habit, so we need to follow the routine of habit formation here as well. You will win new friends and admirers without having to impress them or conform to the pressure of doing things their way. You will be bubbling with life. You will be rearing to go and accomplish all you can with your new found confidence. The best part of adopting the 'positive thinking and a positive attitude of gratitude is that, you will be able to enjoy the smallest pleasures of nature with a heightened sense of satisfaction and awe. We can see and watch a beautiful flower and carry that joy in our mind for future enjoyment with a clear positive habit. We can go back to work freshen and can use it as an object to meditate on when we feel stressed. When we have this attitude, we are able to work without any external pressure to perform but there is sufficient pressure and motivation from within.

The habit of happy living is like any other habit, so we need to follow the routine of habit formation here as well. Happiness is our own choice and decision. Each of us can be as happy as we make up our minds to be. We can, if we want, fill up our days with positive attitude chatter and laughter. To be happy, we need to concentrate only on happy thoughts. The ghosts of the past have to be exorcised. We may be working in any field, the key to success is our outlook. Sometimes we may think that no road is left for us from where you can achieve the happiness of life. There may be chances that someone who was there with us before might hold on to us when we are on the dark side of the life.

Positive thinking and happy living is state of mind.

Positive thinking and happy living is state of mind and happiness is something we cannot earn or buy. We need to remember that people and things alone, won't make us happy. Our own efforts not to get worried or depressed make us happy. Positive living make us happy. We ought to remember the saying, that "Positive living along can bring happiness as it is a state of mind".

The ultimate goal of life should be to get happiness.

The ultimate goal of life should be to get happiness and not get involved into unnecessary worries falling in the death trap of defeats and failures. The essence of life is not in the great victories and grand failures, but in the simple joys. The purpose of our lives is to be happy. Laugh when we can, apologize when we should, and let go of what we can't change. Let us think positive and just visualize that what is stored in destiny would not be negative. If we want to be happy, practice meditation.

If we want, others to be happy practice compassion. Whoever is happy will make others happy, too. Thus we can lead our path to happy sweet and good living.

Our greatest gift to others is to be happy.

Let us be very sure and let us keep in mind that happiness doesn't depend on any superficial conditions, it is governed by our mental attitude only. Our greatest gift to others is to be happy and to radiate our happiness to the entire world. Happiness is a guide to direction, not a place to hide. As a happy person, we radiate happiness to the world. We need to visualize our light radiating throughout the world, passing from person to person until it encircles the globe. Resolve to keep happy, and your joy and you shall form an invincible host against difficulties.

The positive persons often dance to the happy tunes.

The positive persons often dance to the happy tunes of their lives. The path to happiness is forgiveness of everyone and gratitude for everything. Happiness fills your heart each day and your whole life through with clean thoughts. Any day would be a wonderful day if you do not to take life so seriously. Happiness is not about being a winner it is about being gentle with life being gentle within you. Happiness blooms in the presence of self-respect and the absence of ego. Love yourself. Love everyone around you. Love everyone in the whole world.

Happiness is not about being a winner it is about being gentle

When you're feeling depressed or anxious, close your eyes and try to visualize a guided positive imaginary thing. First breathe deeply and relax. How important it is to consistently reach for positive, uplifting, inspirational thoughts. Thought that promote aliveness and abundance. Thoughts that make you feel good. Happiness is not about being a winner it is about being gentle. The only thing between us and our desire, to be happy, is one single fact: we are not happy because we often fall into the death trap of depression and wholly because of our negative thoughts.

Throw away all your negative thoughts.

Throw away all your negative thoughts and worries, concentrate on the goals to be achieved, on the ray of happiness in you and make sure that you are not falling again into the path of negativity. Positive and happy living is not state of mind only it is the discernment of the negatives thoughts .Be a positive thinker and ignore reality in favor of aspirational thoughts. It is more about taking a proactive approach to life. Instead of feeling hopeless or overwhelmed, positive thinking and happy living allows to tackle life's challenges by looking for effective ways to resolve conflict and come up with creative solutions to problems. It might not be easy, but the positive person will surely win and lead a sweet happy and good life.

Happiness in life comes through the doors of positive thoughts;

We do not even realize which one is left open. We have so many reasons to cry and at the same time plenty of reasons to smile as well.

Keeping our dreams and hope alive might be a reason that success and happiness will come our way again. We ought to know that happiness alone does not stand for anything, but it is on our way of thinking that how do we keep ourselves happy in life. Ending up our lives does not lead us to our destination but of course proves we are supposed to be cowards who know not to unfold the doors of belief in God and in ourselves.

Failure and disappointment are part of our life.

Failure and disappointment are part of our life. The only thing is that we need to face them boldly and courageously and try our best to solve the problem. We must not forget to believe in God whatever our situation may be we need to make our faith strong enough not be let down, rather we would break the knees of sorrows and force it to die and lead happy lives. We should not surrender but must find out ways to come out of our worries, anxieties and difficulties. We ought not to indulge ourselves into the darkness of the room but find out the doors to free ourselves from unnecessary fear and worries. We must belief in ourselves and our hearts, and believe in the ones who love us and not the ones whom we love. We must not fall on the negative side of a thing. The experience has taught us that we should buy some strength, hope and positive ness from our loved ones to help ourselves in such a situation rather than surrendering our lives to God as it is a precious gift of God which is equipped with full of joy and happiness we need to help ourselves in these critical moments and live with considerable optimism. Happy living is sure to make our life good and sweet.

It is the real time when you keep on revealing the truth of our lives and relations, do not fall on the reverse side but think how good it was that because of the hard times of our lives we could well judge about them.

We should always try to be positive and happy

We should always try to be positive and should think that whatever is happening, it is the positive side or consequence of that incident in would be on the positive side of our imagination. With all these thoughts, I would request my readers to implement some good thoughts in their life that would make things easier to be tackled by them. We should accept the situation and fight it with more determination.

In this world nothing is good or bad and only thinking makes it so.

We ought to know that advice from people around us will help us to overcome from the any drastic situation. Also we have to always minimize the stress as it gives nothing but takes away joy and happiness from our lives. And finally we need to take things casually and fight with it seriously. A clear minded person looks for good qualities in the other person, whereas a negative mind always looks for the fault in the other person and also a negative mind always looks for the fault. An optimist goes forward keeping in mind the past, a pessimist thinks of the future and reverts back to the past. In fact negative thoughts are our greatest enemies.

Experience the happiness in all circumstances by maintaining better relationships.

Sadness cannot touch a person with a positive attitude. It increases the decision of making power. Creative way of thoughts appears in the mind. Positive thoughts of happy living teach us the art of finding solutions to any problem. Optimism is something what we do. Anxiety and other negative emotions are known to be detrimental to the body, especially to our immune systems, and having an optimistic nature seems to protect against those effects. People who are supposed to be optimistic, about their future, are sure to lead a sweet good and happy life. Their secret of happiness is that they do exercise, do not indulge in in smoking and often follow a good and better diet. Whenever we are unhappy, if we analyze the reason for our unhappiness, it is because life is not matching our expectations.

LEAVE WORRIES NOW BE HAPPY ENJOY LIFE

CHAPTER 7

WORRY-LESS AND GET MORE HAPPINESS

If you are interested in getting more success and happiness within you, focus on all the ways as if you have already attained success. You need to focus on the thing and create a happy live within you. If you want love and affection, focus on all the people and the abundance of love that you have to give to them. If we want to have greater health, focus on all the ways that we are healthy, thus creating and delivering a good life within you. You need to admit that there are problems that you cannot change. But you can change the way of your thinking if you identify the main reason of the problem. And if you acknowledge the facts, that you have been negative or inactive in finding a solution to the problem, probably this will make it easier for you to become positive thus creating a new lease of life within you. It will make your life easier to lead a good and sweet life.

You must try to make goals

You must try to make goals. Making goals can give you a more positive outlook on life. People often tend to get bored with life and get the feeling that they are stuck to negative things which the result they often get the feeling of being depressed. Setting a direction for yourself and a goal would surely help you to move forward.

Mental attitude that can bring you peace and happiness

If you expecting to succeed, and are not afraid of failure, you have the best chance of staying positive and can create a very positive life within you. When you, or any of your associates, are tempted to worry about a problem, write out the solution and a definite answer to it. This helps a positive feeling to generate within you making you very positive to have a good living. Another thing you need to understand is that there are several ways to cultivate a mental attitude that can bring you peace and happiness and can carnage a good life within you. More of it if you fill your mind with thoughts of peace, courage, health, and hope, your life will be easy to live. You would get a happy feeling of life and mind if you let yourself to forget your own unhappiness, by trying to create a little happiness for others. You are best to yourself and to others.

The first step is to write down your worries

The first step is to write down your worries, which will help you make sense of them, and then decide on one small step you can take towards a solution. But to be very true no man in this world is free of obstacles or difficulties. Don't make worry your habit. Break this habit and stop all the negative and panic thoughts provoking your mind all the time. If you can't change the past, but you must not ruin the present by worrying about the future. Joy is what happens to us when we allow ourselves to recognize how good things really are. When we feel worried and depressed, we need to consciously form a smile on our faces and act upbeat until the happy feeling becomes genuine reality.

Happiness is what is needed most.

What makes to lead a happy life is not to get trapped into unnecessary unwanted worries and negative thoughts.

Don't create the feeling of depression and anger. Feelings of depression and hopelessness and or anger are even tougher to cope with on a consistent basis. When you are worried, you not only hurt yourself, but the limited support systems that are still holding on your mind but making you to get more and more worried and nothing is achieved in terms of success except the re-carnation of worries and worries thus leading you to be unhappy and worried all the time. Your actions breed confidence and courage. If you want to conquer fear, anger and worry do not sit ideal and just think about it. Let our deep worrying become advance thinking and planning. If you look into your own mind and heart, and you find nothing wrong there, what is there to worry about? Practically nothing what is there to fear about and again nothing? So why worry unnecessarily and make your present and future dark. Neglect all those which make your life unhappy.

Why being a negative person?

Why being a negative person and what do you get out of it being a depression dejected and sad man.? Why not turn your thoughts to be a positive person simply it is a question of tilting your mind towards a positive side of thing. See both the aspects of a situation and ways the pros and cons of both the sides and try to abolish the negativity in you. Be positive strong and you will remain happy for ever. We all have different roles that we play in the lives of people we love and care about. Our actions and how well we play our part has a direct influence on their life, so we better get in there and give our best performance. Tell them with how much you care in the capacity that you're in. At the end of the day, money is just a means to an end. Nothing more.

If you're grinding and struggling to make ends meet and buried under piles of debt, that's pretty stressful. Once you have your basic needs met though, more money only makes you happier up to a certain point. Money cannot buy you happiness. You need to generate it yourself. Someone will always be better than you at something, but it does not matter. Be inspired by them, using it to push yourself further, and nothing more. If they can do it, why cannot you?

Are you are interested in getting more happiness?.

If you are interested in getting more happiness focus on all the ways as if you have already attained success. You need to focus on the thing and create a live within you. If you want love and affection, focus on all the people and the abundance of love that you have to give to them.

Worrisome thoughts reproduce faster.

Worrisome thoughts reproduce faster so one of the most powerful ways to stop the spiral of worry is simply to disclose the worry to a friend. Practice happy gratitude daily. Take three minutes at the end of your day to chill and write down a small list of the things that can make you smile, laugh, or that you're glad are a part of your life. There's something to be grateful about, especially when you look down at that list and realize that a lot of people have it worse off than you do and could use a few of those things. Simply being an optimist will not solve all your problems, but what's the alternative is to keep your mind and heart cool and always have happy and positive feeling and think that life is to live happily. There isn't much sense in being anything else.

If you're constantly filling your head with negative thoughts, odds are they'll lead you straight towards negative actions, self-doubt and increase the general happiness of life isn't a cool place to live at all. Think of each setback as a challenge to see the positive, spin the situation back around, making it better than it was before and start living in a good and sweet manner.

What do we get out of unhappiness?

We may feel largely uncomfortable, when worries attack our thoughts and mind. While we are consuming more worries we are far too busy to do anything else to fix the real problem and would rather find it hard to get into a smart solution. Thus resulting in a fact that you spend your evenings worrying only without even bothering to find some time to know its cause. We get nothing out of worrying except only to think and cry and become unhappy. We do not get anything out of unhappiness. Another thing is that we may feel largely uncomfortable, when worries attack our thoughts and mind which makes worrying about a situation an easier option to get depressed and diffused. While we are consuming more worries we are far too busy to do anything else to fix the real problem and would rather find it hard to get into a smart solution. Thus resulting in a fact that we spend our evenings worrying only without even bothering to find some time to search a sweet happiness within us.Negative thought which are provoking our mind, about the uncertainties and the negativities, as to what will happen tomorrow creates unnecessary worries and worries are repetitive thoughts associated with feelings of anxiety in anticipation of some negative future event which may end in a failure.

Negative thoughts create unnecessary worries

Whether the worries are about financial crisis, family problems, work, health or any topic of concern, the anxious feelings and negative thoughts produced are always distinctly unpleasant thus making us unhappy all the time. We get nothing being a negative and unhappy man. We must not forget that if we tend to worry they will never rob tomorrow of its sorrows, but will only deny today of its meaning happiness and joys. Negative thoughts only produce worries and worrying is actually a form of superstition and creates false images in our mind and that is the main reason and cause which makes and leads us to this point of imagination. A human being can survive almost anything, as long as he or she sees the end in sight, starts analyzing his positive thoughts and starts analyzing his unhappiness.

We need to fore see the coming trouble first.

We must not forgot that if something bad or good is to happen it is sure to happen, whether we worry or not. Let us put our energy into today and stop worrying about the future and past. We should not foresee trouble, or worry about what may never happen as past is dead and gone forever and future is uncertain and yet to come. Positive thinking our brave attitude and our courage will ward off everything and bring happiness in our lives. The basic facts we should know about worry. The basic techniques to analyze worry and how to break the worry habit before it breaks us. These are the simple ways where we can concentrate and get rid of worries prevailing in our thoughts, remove all the negativity in our live and start living a positive good and happy life.

Think of good and positive ways of Happy Living.

Annalise positive ways of happy living and get to see the reasons and facts of worry. To avoid reoccurrence of worries, concentrate on prayers as prayers are the best source of remedies of the prevailing worries. Think good ways of living and starting praying. The more you pray, the less you'll panic. The more you worship, the less you worry. There is nothing that wastes the body like worry, and anyone who has any faith in God should need not to worry about anything whatsoever is to happen in future. Positive thinking is the creation of good imagination and good imagination is the creation of sweet and happy living.

Happiness comes with Positive living and sweet thoughts

If you know that the circumstance is beyond your control or power change than revise it to your liking. Just try to put a stop-less order on your worries. Don't permit little things which become insects of life to ruin your happiness. Co-operate with the inevitable. Decide just how much anxiety a thing may be worth and refuse to give in anymore.

All the happiness is not given in one go it comes slowly and slowly with positive thinking.

Have worry under your control. If your worries center around, pay special attention to remain positive and be happy. Keep yourself happy, treat your worried thoughts as valuable signals. How to keep from worrying about criticism? Simply unjust criticism and think positively and do often discard a bad compliment. It often means that you have aroused jealousy and envy. Let's keep a record of the fool things we have done and stop criticizing ourselves.

Cause of unhappiness is Negative way of living life

The utmost cause of worry is our negative thinking as it leads us to the state of depression. Living will change for the better-If You Think Positive. Our negative thinking and attitude towards suffering and depression becomes very important because it can affect how we cope with suffering when it arises. Depression is nourished by a lifetime of un-grieved and unforgiven causes. Times will change for the better when you change. Worry is a misuse of the imagination. Worry is most often a prideful way of thinking that you have more control over life and its circumstances than you actually do. Positive Thinking leads your way to good and happiness. An art of Good and Happy Living.

Neglect worries keep yourself happy.

Neglect worries keep yourself happy, treat your worried thoughts as valuable signals. These are the fundamental facts you should be familiar about worries. A huge factor to stay happy is to cater your worries around, an important relationship in your life and pay special attention sustaining positive relationships. Worries are there to motivate information gathering and problem-solving. Make your mind firm and do come to a positive decision as come what we will not allow the worries to entire our mind and soul.

What if we just acted like everything was easy?

Once a decision is carefully reached we should get busy carrying out our decisions and should not bother about all the anxieties that are about to come. When we, or any of our colleagues or associates, are about to worry about a problem, we must write it out and think positively of the questions.

Instead of worrying about what people say of you, why not spend time trying to accomplish something they will admire. What if we just acted like everything was easy? How would your life be different if you stopped worrying about things we can't control and started focusing on the things we can? Let today be the day. Free yourself from fruitless worry, seize the day and take effective action on things you can change. We would change ourselves for the betterment if we start thinking in positive terms. Positive thinking is what is required of us and simply worrying about the future things or as to what will happen in the next moment will certainly deprive us of good and happy living that we are about gather or get in the next hour.

Another cause of getting worried or unhappy is the attachment

Attachment brings worry. If you have a problem and you come up with the answer, you stop worrying immediately. Our minds can be dishonest, persuading us that we are worrying about something, when our deepest fear is entirely different. No-one likes to admit that they've chosen to worry.

The first step is to write down your worries, which will help you make sense of them, and then decide on one small step you can take towards a solution. But to be very true no man in this world is free of obstacles or difficulties. Don't make worry your habit. Break this habit and stop all the negative and panic thoughts provoking your mind all the time if you want to remain a happy person and lead a happy good and sweet life. Feelings of depression and angry are even tougher to cope with on a consistent basis.

When you are worried, you not only hurt yourself, but the limited support systems that are still holding on your mind making you to get more and more worried and nothing is achieved in terms of success except the re-carnation of worries and worries Joy is what happens to us when we allow ourselves to recognize how good things really are.

Practically nothing what is there to fear about?

So why worry unnecessarily and make your present and future dark. Why being a negative person and what do you get out of it being a depression dejected and sad man.? Why not turn your thoughts to be a positive person simply it is a question of tilting your mind towards a positive side of thing. See both the aspects of a situation and ways the pros and cons of both the sides and try to abolish the negativity in you. You will surely be a happy man.

Think of the best the best is sure to happen

Think of the best the best is sure to happen and if you think of the worst the worst will come. Better come forward wake up and think positive first. Positive persons always succeed in life whatever be the circumstances and the negative often dig a death trap for themselves. So why be a negative person why you have all the qualities of being a positive man. Surround yourself with friends and people that are better than you in areas that you want to improve in.

LEAVE WORRIES NOW
BE HAPPY ENJOY LIFE

CHAPTER 8

BE BOLD AND HAVE POSITIVE THINKING

If you are interested in getting more happiness, focus on all the ways as if you have already attained success. You need to focus on the thing and create a live within you. Positive thinking will generate happiness in you. Our actions positive thinking breed confidence and courage in us. If we want to conquer fear, anger and worry we should sit ideal and just think about it. Let our deep worrying do some advance thinking and planning. If we look into our own mind and heart, and we will find nothing wrong there, what is there to worry about and generate unhappiness in us?

Is there anything to be unhappy about?

Practically nothing what is there to be unhappy about? So why worry unnecessarily and make our present and future dark. Discard negative thought think positive and be happy. Positive thinking is the key to all problems and worries. Solve all your problems and get rid of all unnecessary worries by simply thinking in a positive manner. What is there to worry about? Think positive, be positive and have confidence in you. You will create great happiness within yourself. You need to admit that there are problems that you cannot change. But you can change the way of your thinking if you identify the main reason of the problem.

And if you acknowledge the facts, that you have been negative or inactive in finding a solution to the problem, probably this will make it easier for you to become positive thus creating a new lease of life within you.

You must try to make goals.

Making goals can give you a more positive outlook on life. People often tend to get bored with life and get the feeling that they are stuck to negative things which the result they often get the feeling of being depressed. Setting a direction for yourself and a goal would surely help you to move forward. If you expecting to succeed, and are not afraid of failure, you have the best chance of staying positive and can create a very positive life within you.

When you, or any of your associates, are tempted to worry about a problem, write out the solution and a definite answer to it. This helps a positive feeling to generate within you. Another thing you need to understand is that there are several ways to cultivate a mental attitude that can bring you peace and happiness and can carnage a good life within you.

There are several ways to cultivate a mental attitude.

More of it if you fill your mind with thoughts of peace, courage, health, and hope, your life will be easy to live. You would get a happy feeling of life and mind if you let yourself to forget your own unhappiness, by trying to create a little happiness for others. You are best to yourself. The perfect way to conquer worry is the Prayer of God.

To keep yourself from worrying about criticism, do not even try to get mixed with your enemies, because if you do you will hurt yourself far more than we hurting them. Instead of worrying about ingratitude, let's expect it. Let's remember that the only way to find happiness is not to expect gratitude, but to give for the joy of giving. Let us build a happy life within us generate peace and a healthy atmosphere around us.

Let us build a happy life within us

This will help us to lead a peaceful happy and prosperous life and we would find ourselves to be happier than before. You should do things in the order of their importance. You need to clear your desk of all papers except those relating to the immediate problem at hand. When you face a problem, solve it then and there, if you have the facts to make a decision.

Make a decision fast and do not linger on. Learn to organize, deputize, and supervise and straight away come to decision. Simply postponing it would spoil your good thoughts and there is every likelihood your mind may get into negative activities and start thinking in negative manner. Therefore write down a list of things that make you excited, however big, small, likely or unlikely. Then work to make them occur more often. Look for moments of joy and savor them. Recognize your good happening every day.

Eat well do plenty of exercise and do not skip meals.

It is a known fact that physical exercise is known to stimulate our veins and get to strengthen our minds that lift depression and anxiety so we need to walk, swim, run or whatever we like doing best. Those who create or those who do well on the worst scenario, give themselves worry and stress, tend to be devastated. If we cannot get some sunshine, we can always lighten up our rooms with brighter lights.

We can have lunch outside the office. Take frequent walks instead of driving our cars over short distances. No man is indispensable. First of all our circle of friends is always there to give us some moral support. Spending time and engaging ourselves in worthwhile activities could give us a very enjoyable and satisfying feeling. Nothing feels better than having group support.

Good friends are quite important and their company generally lightened up our spirits. To get to know and to find such friends we simply have to be friendly with ourselves, and then the friendships will naturally follow us. We need to understand the power of touch and support and we have not to underestimate it strength and support. Don't we feel so good when someone pats us on our back and gives us some words of encouragement during your most challenging times and difficult times? Just hug or embrace someone someday you will see that you have almost changed his life. Get intimate with him and try to establish close ties with his family and friends. The love and care expressed by you will tremendously boost him and well as your immune system and fury of worry will be diminished for all.

In our lives storms may come and go. In the form of reversals, but if we have the power and foundation of inner fulfillment and if we deal with it with a very clear practical mind these storms will not kill us or will not disrupt us. There could be numberless reasons for which we keep on worrying. We may be worried about our health, wealth, loved ones, friends, the happening of yesterday and the follow happenings of tomorrow, the environment or the world politics, but these can be dealt with firm mind and fearless worry if we generate within ourselves the power of enlightenment within ourselves. There's no sense in worrying about the negatives if these negatives cannot be changed. If we waste energy and happiness on the things we can't change, we'll only make ourselves more frustrated and come to the stage of depression dejection and disappointments.

Negativity is a habit.

Negativity is a habit and we often don't realize we're doing ourselves down. Under each negative thought that we have written, we can spot an alternative way of looking at it, that isn't so negative.

Take your mind to positivity and mold and drive your thoughts to the positivity. There's a world of difference between expecting failure or rejection so as not to be disappointed when it occurs and recognizing it as a possibility of being positive. It's sensible to look at a situation from all angles and to have a back-up plan to fall back on if need be.

People who do this will not see failure as another step on the road to eventual success; but by expecting and envisioning success, there's less likely to be a failure. Let us find some ways of removing negative thoughts and discouraging our worries to be born.

Let us all generate and create happiness within us

Let us all generate and create happiness within us by removing all negative thoughts negative feeling and unwanted desires that make our mind greedy and spoil the charm of our sweet good and happy living.

LEAVE WORRIES NOW
BE HAPPY ENJOY LIFE

CHAPTER 9

NEGATIVE THINKING CAN RUIN YOUR LIFE

Remember three aspects - naturalness, simplicity and belongingness. Just open up your heart and be natural. Next is living a simple life. Living with the confidence will get whatever is needed, that is simplicity. Right or wrong, we are what we are. We need to tone our life accordingly and if we live like this naturally, then there will not be any fear. There will be no doubts or blocks in life. This is the important mantra of Art of Sweet Living. Another important thing is that if we cannot get some good sunshine, we can always lighten up our thoughts with brighter lights of happy living. We can have ample of lunch of positive thinking. To avoid negative thoughts we need to take frequent walks. No man is indispensable and no man is not capable of positive thinking. Let us make ourselves happy and life become a sweet living.

Happiness is a state of mind.

We know the saying, that "Happiness is a state of mind". And state of mind is what we think and what we do or act in a peaceful manner without being getting worried or depressed. If you are interested in getting more happiness, to get it through positive thinking. All we need to do is to focus on all the directions on positive thinking and happy living as if we have already attained success. We need to focus on the thing and create a life within us.

If we want love and affection, entertain people and give them the abundance of love. If we want to have greater health, pay attention on all the ways that make us healthy, thus creating and delivering a good life within us by thinking in positive ways. We need to understand and admit that there are problems that we cannot change. But we can change the ways of our thinking and if we identify the main reason of the problem we can remove all the obstacles coming in our way of leading a sweet and happy life. And if we acknowledge the fact, that we have been negative or inactive in finding a solution to the problem, this will make it easier for us to become positive thus creating a new lease of life within us.

Positive thinking will surely make us happy.

Another thing to understand is that we must try to make our goals. Making goals can give us a more positive outlook on life. People often tend to get bored with life and get the feeling that they are stuck to negative things with the result they often get the feeling of being depressed dejected and monotonous and become unhappy in life. Setting a direction and a goal for ourselves, would surely help us to move forward. If we are expecting to succeed, and are not afraid of failure, we stand the best chance of staying positive and thus can create a very positive life within us.

Mental attitude that can bring you peace and happiness.

Another thing you need to understand is that there are several ways to cultivate a mental attitude that can bring you peace and happiness and can carnage a good life within you.

More of it if you fill your mind with thoughts of peace, courage, health, and hope, your life will be easy to live. If you think in positive terms you would get a happy feeling of life and mind you if you let yourself to forget your own unhappiness, by trying to create a little happiness for others you are sure to get happiness in your live. You are best to yourself. The perfect way to conquer worry is the Prayer of God. You should do things in the order of their importance.

Learn to think in positive terms.

When you face a problem, solve it then and there, by thinking positively and if you have the facts of making a decision, make a decision fast and do not linger on. Learn to think in positive terms organize the things, deputise, and supervise straight away by coming to decision. To keep yourself from worrying about criticism, do not even try to get mixed with your enemies, because if you do you will hurt yourself far more than we hurting them. You will fall prey to negative thinking and this in turn will lead you unhappiness in life. Simply postponing it would spoil your good thoughts and there is every likelihood your mind may get into negative activities and start thinking in negative manner. Therefore think positive, write down a list of things that make you positive, however big, small, likely or unlikely. Then work to make them occur more often. Look for moments of joy and savor them. Recognise your good happening every day. Be positive think positive and be happy.

Happiness is your own choice and decision

You may also feel that life has become terrible for you to live and you are carrying no hope that someone would be there to rescue you. Happiness is your own choice and decision. Each of us can be as happy as we make up our minds to be. We can, if we want, fill up our days with positive attitude chatter and laughter. To be happy, we need to concentrate only on happy thoughts. Our friends are always there to give us some moral support.

Spending time and engaging ourselves in worthwhile positive activities could give us a very enjoyable and satisfying feeling. Nothing feels better than having group support and talking in terms of positive thinking. Good friends are quite important and their company generally lightened up our spirits. This makes us to think in positive manner and to get to know such friends we simply have to be friendly with ourselves, and then the friendships will naturally follow us and make our lives happy.

Only way to find happiness is not to expect gratitude.

Let us remember that the only way to find happiness is not to expect gratitude, but to give for the joy of giving. Let us build a happy life within us generate peace and a healthy atmosphere around us.

This will help us to lead a peaceful happy and prosperous life and we would find ourselves to be happier than before. We need to understand the power of positive thinking and its support and we have not to underestimate it strength and support.

Don't we feel so good when someone pats us on our back and gives us some words of encouragement during your most challenging times and difficult times and advises us to remain positive and think positive just hug or embrace someone with positive attitude someday we will see that we have almost changed our life. The ghosts of the past have to be exorcised. We may be working in any field, the key to success is our outlook. Sometimes we may think that no road is left for us from where we can achieve the happiness of life. One need not to forgot that we need to eat well do plenty of exercise and do not skip meals It is a known fact that physical exercise is known to stimulate our veins and get to strengthen our minds that lift depression and anxiety, so we need to walk, swim, run or whatever we like doing best above all we must move ahead in direction where our mind can generate electricity to think in positive directly and bring immense happiness to us

Difficulties and storms may come and go.

In our lives difficulties and storms may come and go in the form of reversals, but if we have the power of positive thinking and foundation of inner fulfillment we would be able to deal with it with a very clear practical mind and with this positive thinking these storms will not kill us nor will disrupt us. There could be numberless reasons for which we keep on worrying. We may be worried about our health, wealth, loved ones, friends, the happening of yesterday and the follow happenings of tomorrow, the environment or the world politics, but these can be dealt with firm mind and fearless worry.

If we generate within ourselves the power of positive thinking within ourselves and try to be happy all the time.

The best thing about happiness is that we get it is free.

We don't have to pay or we do not have to open any account to be happy. We don't have to pay monthly rent for it either. We just have to change our perspective, our views on what we are seeing and feeling. Happiness is not something which is quite readymade. It comes from our own actions and deeds.

Angriness and happiness don't mix.

We must dig out the angriness in us, and see that the happiness has shown and seeded a place to grow its roots. The ultimate goal of life should be to get happiness and not get involved into unnecessary worries falling in the death trap of defeats and failures. The essence of life is not in the great victories and grand failures, but in the simple joys. The purpose of our lives is to be happy.

If you want to be happy, be positive first practice meditation.

Laugh when you can, apologize when you should, and let go of what you can't change. Think positive and just visualize that what is stored in destiny would not be negative. If you want to be happy, be positive first practice meditation. If you want, others to be happy practice compassion. Whoever is happy will make others happy, too.

Happiness doesn't depend on any superficial conditions.

Let us be very sure and let us keep in mind that happiness doesn't depend on any superficial conditions, it is governed by our mental attitude only. Our greatest gift to others is to be happy and to radiate our happiness to the entire world. Happiness is a guide to direction, not a place to hide. As a happy person, we radiate happiness to the world.

We need to visualise our light radiating throughout the world, passing from person to person until it encircles the globe. Resolve to keep happy, and you shall form an invincible host against difficulties.

The path to happiness is forgiveness.

The positive persons often dance to the happy tunes of their lives. The path to happiness is forgiveness of everyone and gratitude for everything. Happiness fills our heart each day and our whole life through with clean thoughts. Any day would be a wonderful day if we do not to take life so seriously. Happiness is not about being a winner it is about being gentle with life being gentle within us. Happiness blooms in the presence of self-respect and the absence of ego. Love yourself.

Love everyone around you. Love everyone in the whole world. When you're feeling depressed or anxious, close your eyes and try to visualize a guided positive imaginary thing. First breathe deeply and relax. How important it is to consistently reach for positive, uplifting, inspirational thoughts. Thought that promote aliveness and abundance. Thoughts that make you feel good. Imagine that you are already a positive person and you love life.

The only thing between us and our desire, to be happy, is one single fact: we are not happy because we often fall into the death trap of depression and wholly because of our negative thoughts. Absence of positive thinking, has eluded us of our great happiness and left us far behind. This very little known fact has kept many of us from reaching our goal of happiness. Throw away all your negative thoughts and worries, concentrate on the goals to be achieved, on the ray of happiness in you and make sure that you are not falling again into the path of negativity.

Happiness can only be achieved if you have a positive mind.

Happiness is a state of mind only and not the thoughts of negatives, and it quite true that happiness can only be achieved if you have a positive mind and a clear attitude of being a positive person. Happiness and positivity go hand in hand. If you are positive you are a happy person and if you possess negativity you would land yourself to be a very negative person thus ruining your life for what of nothing with the result you become an unhappy person and you remain aloof from leading a sweet good and happy living.

LEAVE WORRIES NOW
BE HAPPY ENJOY LIFE

CHAPTER 10

STEPS FOR GOOD AND HAPPY LIFE

It might not be easy, but the positive impact it will have on our mental, emotional, and physical health will be well-worth it .At time we may think that there is no road is left for us from where we can achieve the happiness of our lives. We may also feel that life has become terrible for us to live and we are carrying new hope that someone would come to rescue us. There may be chances that someone who was there with us before might have held on to us when we were on the dark side of the life.

Life itself is a stage and we all are the performers.

What if when everything goes wrong and all the doors of happiness are closed our live becomes a silent. It is a quite common and we are aware of a marvelous proverb that Life itself is a stage and we all are the performers, performing different acts assigned to us by our almighty power. We should not forget as to what is in our possession, if it is to fulfill our duties towards our responsibility and do whatever is correct and is allowed by us in our life? We should not forget that happiness in life comes through the doors of positive thoughts; we need to have them first. If one door happen to close, another opens, in the event only when we are confident and optimistic. We have so many reasons to cry and at the same time plenty of reasons to smile as well.

Similarly, happiness does not stand for anything, but is on our way of thinking that how do we keep ourselves happy in life. Failure and disappointment are part of our life. The only thing is that we need to face and solve the problem is by keeping our dreams and hope alive be it a reason that success and happiness will come our way again.

Smiling and the doubt free character which is the foremost important reason for a successful and happy life.

There are quite a number of reasons to believe that for a successful and happy life the mystery surrounding it lies in our interests, and good memory which is the basis of our interest, power of desire and aim, keeping ourselves smiling and the doubt free character which is the foremost important reason for a successful and happy life. If we possess one solid unselfish and doubt free character within ourselves we would be quite happy and successful. The experience has taught us that we should buy some strength, hope and positivity from our loved ones to help ourselves in such a situation rather than surrendering as life is a precious gift of God and is equipped with full of joy and happiness if we help ourselves in these critical moments we can live with considerable optimism. Now let's us imagine that we are not feeling at our best today, and we are having thoughts that could be classified as negative. We shouldn't be thinking such negative thoughts. We don't like the negative thoughts. We ought to know that negative thoughts are stressful, demoralizing and depressing. We shouldn't aim to have negative thoughts at all.

Often we feel uncomfortable because we think we have to say or do something in response to another person's words. When we find ourselves thinking this way, it helps enormously to take a few moments to check inside and notice what we are feeling. We are deeply depressed that negativity has governed us and has taken a deep root in our minds. So, let's imagine that you have chosen to focus on your negative thinking with regards to school.

Evaluating thoughts can generate happiness within us.

The next step is to spend a little bit of time each day evaluating your own thoughts. When you find yourself thinking critical thoughts about yourself, take a moment to pause and reflect. While you might be upset about getting a bad grade on an exam, is berating yourself really the best approach? Is there any way to put a positive spin on the situation?

While you might not have done well on this exam, at least you have a better indication of how to structure your study time for the next big test. However, despite of all these good thoughts which are embodied to us by the almighty fail to revive these unwanted circumstances that lead us to sorrow and difficulties and a situation where we do not know what is correct and good for us and what is wrong for us.

Life is there, where there is hope.

We should always remember that, "Life is there, where there is hope".

That single thing that remains in our hands is to find out ways to know how to overcome these worries of our life at that very moment when all doors are closed for us which means that whatever situation is there, we must not give up hope. We must fight because there have been always a chance that with good faith and hard work we can turn the odds in our favor. It is often said that it is very easy to advice but when it comes to us, things go out of our control and we fail to suggest a way out for ourselves.

Happy living allows us to tackle life's challenges

We fall into the trap of unnecessary worries and elope ourselves with negative thoughts. We feel better when somebody else is facing some difficulty but when it comes to us we fail to gather that faith, will power and the words of strength. Being a positive thinker is not about ignoring reality in favor of aspirational thoughts. It is more about taking a proactive approach to our lives. Instead of feeling hopeless or overwhelmed, positive thinking allows us to tackle life's challenges by looking for effective ways to resolve conflict and come up with creative solutions to problems. It might not be easy, but the positive impact it will have on our mental, emotional, and physical health will be well-worth it. It takes practice; lots of practice. This is not a step-by-step process that we can complete and be done with. Instead, it involves a lifelong commitment to looking inside ourselves and being willing to challenge negative thoughts and make positive changes. It is a common fact that no one in this world is free of obstacles or difficulties.

If all the openings of happiness are shut for us and we have to overcome that and have no way to come out, but to survive lest we must have to learn to swim out of the sorrows because this is what is called life and sorrow free living. There are lot more examples and in many other situations, where we will find that how we could have faced and fought with our sorrows and difficulties of life when there was no hope left in our lives. As commonly said by big saints that the self- seeking man who is looking after his personal comforts and leading a lazy life for himself there would be no room for him even in the hell and he simply have lost the power of his will and he cannot lead a happy life.

The secret of every successful man is to have, good confidence

The secret of every successful man is to have, good confidence, faith and strength behind him and that remain the right cause of his single success in life. Unselfishness plays a very vital role in his life. He may not have been perfectly unselfish, yet he was tending towards it. If he had been perfectly unselfish, he would have been as great a success.

The degree of unselfishness marks the degree of success everywhere and he leads to be successful man without fear worries and selfishness. Therefore creation of positivity in life is utmost necessary to enjoy the special gift of God to us. The love for God and worshipping God adds to one common thing the immense faith in Him.

There may be different beliefs and ways to worship God in different communities, places and religions, but one thing remains the same and that is the Love of God for all of us. Our world is full of odds and evens, happiness and sorrows, fulfilment and emptiness. And these are all created by the Almighty. However, the most beautiful Gift of God, is Human, which is such a mystery driven by Him which could hardly be defined or explained in depth.

If aim of our life is to stay happy and let others to be happy, we will be happy and remembered by all.

We know that life cannot be foreseen. Life is not a bed of roses. Life is a battle field and not a bed of roses as every man on earth has to struggle very hard in making his life happy. But no one will actually remember us for the wealth we have gained, or success we have achieved until and unless we do not live a happy life. Life is such a special gift of Almighty and it is not gifted by Him to use it the way we like or love to. The actual path shown by Him needs to be followed by us for us to reach the peak of betterment every moment. We need to have some positive attitude to look at it comfortably but at the same time having a positive mental attitude does not mean banishing all negative thoughts and people from your life. We need to believe that a positive attitude is a choice. This step is hard to take. People are either positive or negative. They tend to blame their negativity on all kinds of outside forces fate, experiences, parents, relationship, but never really stopped to think that they could choose to be positive. Piercing ourselves that positivity is a choice has been one of the greatest things we have ever done for ourselves.

Now when we find ourselves in a bad situation, we know that it's up to us to find the good, to be positive regardless of what's happening around us. We should no longer point fingers and place blame to anyone else. We need to realize that everything happens how it happens, and it's up to us to choose how we want to feel about it. We need to be in control of our attitude, and no one can take that away this from us. If we want to live a positive, joyful and happy life, we must not be surrounded by negative people who don't encourage our happiness. As a negative person, we ought to get attracted too negative people only. Only when we decide to make the change to live a more positive life, we have to get rid of our lives of the most negative influences in it. We are quite aware of the fact that no one is perfect and perfection isn't the goal when it comes to positivity but there were people in our lives who were consistently negative, who constantly bring us down, we need to stop spending so much time with them.

We can very well imagine, it is not easy for us to get away from these negative people.

It can hurt us to keep distance from people even when you know they aren't good for us and for our current lifestyle. In addition to removing negative influences from them, we also have to get rid of some of our own negative behaviors, such as the drug and alcohol abuse. We need to take some concrete steps and examine which behaviors are good for us and which were not harmful. What we need is to learn to focus on the positive things, such as working on positive activities and cultivating new, positive relationships. We must let go of the negative ones.

This process may be not easy to live a positive life when negative people and behaviors continually pull us down. In every situation or in every person there is something good. Most of the time it's not easy to find the positive qualities but we have to look hard to discover positivity in them. Now, when we are faced with a difficult or challenging situation, we need to think and talk to ourselves and console our mind, no matter how terrible the situation might seem, we can always find something good if we take the time to think about it.

Anything good and bad is learning experience.

It is quite obvious that anything good and bad is learning experience so, at the very least, we must learn from bad experiences. However, there's usually even more to it than that. If you really take some time to have a look at it, we would find something good, something genuinely positive, about every person or situation. Not only do we need to be happy with ourselves for this multiple action to take effect, but we also need to be more positive and happy with others. We have to share our wealth of happiness with the people of the world. The best way is to be nice with other people, no matter what. Tell them that they look nice today. Appreciate their job and tell them that have done a great job on that assignment. Be happy and tell your elder or your kids how much you love them and how great they are. When someone is feeling down, do what we need to do is to cheer him or her up. Do send them gifts nice flower and glow them with nice notes. By doing this we will not make ourselves happy but in turn give and generate happiness for others too.

At times we may suffer from chronic depression, though we know how good things look on to others life cannot be worse for us. Let's imagine how to deal when life leaves a great big steaming pile at our doorstep. Lest we need to remember that external factors can be dealt with by taking positive and happy steps to repair or at least address the root of the problem as best as we can. Whatever may be the primary cause of the problem, that cause must be examined first? What is required is that we never wanted to see the good in ourselves and, therefore, didn't want to see it in others also. We must not be critical and condescending rather we must be encouraging and supportive. We should not try to treat others as we would like to be treated, but also try to consider how we would like to be treated. The world likes to appreciate positivity, and the more we share it with others, the more we would be practicing it your own lives. When we start feeling like the idea of not being a happy person we need to remind ourselves that all it takes is one tiny step in the right direction to move towards a more happy life.

Share your happy thoughts with others

We have to believe in ourselves and remember the most important lesson of all is a happy outlook and that is a choice that we can always make. The power of remaining happy, whatever the situation, can never be underestimated. We are all here for a short duration, but is it worth it to spend any of that time in a any angry or being negative? That need to sort out in mind and soul and thus must share our happy thoughts with others.

The real test of any one is to remain happy whenever some challenges become difficult. Remaining happy keeps our mind in the right state of balance and often opens resolutions to the problems at hand. Negativity is contagious and spreads like fire. It not only does its affect anyone, but it spreads to everyone who ever comes in contact with it or whoever they interact with. When only the negative perspective is in focus, the resolution process is impeded. Eliminating negativity, or rather, being positive is a mindset that can be found at any moment, and which can be turned into a habit. We must throw away the negativity in us and opt for being a very positive person this in turn will make us happy and we would be able to lead a sweet and happy life forever.

The secret of successful and happy life lies in keeping ourselves smiling

We need to learn a lesson from every situation. No matter how difficult the situation may appear. We should recognize the beautiful lessons waiting to be discovered. Sometimes lessons may prove to be expensive and costly, but every problem is a learning experience in disguise. We need to be conscious of our thoughts, especially, when life just isn't going our way. The moment we see that we are diving into frustration, agony, sorrow or low self –esteem we must shift our thoughts, by thinking about something completely different and unrelated. You are essentially trying to cultivate a new habit here, the secret of successful and happy life lies in keeping ourselves smiling and the character which is the foremost important reason that lies within us.

Whenever your mind is tempted to jump the fence and start to worry, say this verse aloud or to yourself. You may even have to repeat it over and over again. Am I constantly striving to see the positive in every aspect of my life? Steps for a successful and happy life.

MAKE YOUR WAY TO HAPPY LIVING

We need to believe that a happy living is a matter of our choice. This step is hard to take. People are either positive or negative. They tend to blame their negativity on all kinds of outside forces fate, experiences, parents, relationship, but never really stopped to think that they could choose to be happy. Piercing ourselves that happiness is a choice has been one of the greatest things we have ever done for ourselves. Now when we find ourselves in a bad situation, we know that it is up to us to find the good, to be happy regardless of what is happening around us. We should no longer point fingers and place blame to anyone else. We need to realise that everything happens how it happens, and it is up to us to choose how we want to feel about it. We need to be in control of our attitude and happiness, and no one can take that away this from us.

LEAVE WORRIES NOW
BE HAPPY ENJOY LIFE
CHAPTER 11

UNHAPPINESS IS CONTAGIOUS -

It not only does its affect anyone, but it spreads to everyone who ever comes in contact with it or whoever they interact with. When only the negative perspective is in focus, the resolution process is impeded. Eliminating unhappiness, or rather, being happy is a mindset that can be found at any moment, and which can be turned into a habit. If we want to live a happy, joyful life, we must not be surrounded by negative people who don't encourage our happiness. As a negative person, we ought to get attracted to negative people only. Only when we decide to make the change to live a more positive and happy life, we have to get rid of our lives of the most negative influences in it. We are quite aware of the fact that no one is perfect and perfection is not the goal when it comes to positivity but there were people in our lives who were consistently negative, who constantly bring us down, we need to stop spending so much time with them. We can very well imagine, it is not easy for us to get away from these unhappy people. It can hurt us to keep distance from people even when you know they are not good for us and for our current lifestyle. In addition to removing negative influences from them, we also have to get rid of some of our own negative behaviors, such as the drug and alcohol abuse. We need to take some concrete steps and examine which behaviors are good for us and which were not harmful.

What we need is to learn to focus on the happy things, such as working on positive activities and cultivating new, positive relationships. We must let go of the negative ones. This process may be not easy to live a positive life when negative people and behaviors continually pull us down. We need to discard all of them to lead a happy and sweet life. An art of sweet living lies below us we have only to recognize it.

Look For Sweet Living in Life

The real test of any one is to remain happy whenever some challenges become difficult. Remaining happy keeps our mind in the right state of balance and often opens resolutions to the problems at hand. We must throw away the unhappiness in us and opt for being a very positive person. In every situation or in every person there is something good. Most of the time it's not easy to find the happiness qualities but we have to look hard to discover happiness in them. Now, when we are faced with a difficult or challenging situation, we need to think and talk to ourselves and console our mind, no matter how terrible the situation might seem, we can always find something good if we take the time to think about it. It is quite obvious that anything good and bad is learning experience so, at the very least, we must learn from bad experiences. However, there is usually even more to it than that. If you really take some time to have a look at it, we would find something good, something genuinely happy, about every person or situation. We must look for sweet living in life

Get Sweet feeling in your life

Once we start thinking more in a happy manner, we will
realize that we had to reinforce these thoughts and
behaviors within ourselves so that we could stick to it. As
with any sort of training, the more we practice, the better
we get to be happy. The best and easiest way to do this is to
be happy when it comes to who we are. We need to speak
to ourselves that we are awesome. And we have done a
good job at work thus creating happiness within us. We
need to be honest with ourselves, and we need to do our
best to look for the good. And, whatever we do, we must
not focus on the negative. It is alright not to like everything
about ourselves, but don not focus on what we do not like.
We have all to get the sweet feeling in our lives, and it is up
to us to remind ourselves of them every day.

Share sweet and happy thoughts

Not only do we need to be happy with ourselves for this
multiple action to take effect, but we need to be more
happy with others too.. We have to share our wealth of
happiness with the people of the world. The best way is to
be nice with other people and to make them happy, no
matter what the matter is. Tell them that they look nice
today. What is required is that we never wanted to see the
good in ourselves and, therefore, didn't want to see it in
others also. We must not be critical and condescending
rather we must be encouraging and supportive. We should
not try to treat others as we would like to be treated, but
also try to consider how we would like to be treated. This
will strangle the pattern of self-pity, mind-created
imaginations, and negative downward stairs.

Really what makes us different from other mammals is our ability to control our thoughts and think for ourselves happiness and shift our unhappy thoughts to a happy feelings and to happy living. We may have made mistakes, but now we can accept it and continue, knowing that we will make a different decision in the future. If we understand this it can be appreciative for the experience. We cannot be both angry and grateful at the same time. We should start counting the blessings and miracles in our lives and if we start exploring for them and we would find more happiness in doing so.

Feeling good about ourselves and showing self-confidence.

Feeling good about ourselves and showing self-confidence boosts our skills potential and capabilities in any areas of work and supports us to become happier. We need to shift our thoughts from being a unhappy person to more strong and positive man. Also keeping in mind that pushing things to the limit and going beyond what we think is possible for us to get to the next step of being happy. It becomes another key to achieving what we really want to do. We only want happiness and want to lead a happy life. Even if it may even be relationships and we are finding it difficult to meet someone where we are actually interested in, we need not wait because it usually doesn't come to us by own, we must stand up to get help from any learned fellow. One of the most important things while doing all of this is to be happy about what we are doing, thus we ought to have a successful goal setting our lifestyle with a happy attitude.

We may or may not be able to solve the problem of unhappiness that lies within us, but at least knowing that we are taking positive steps that can help us improve our happiness. It will not be easy, of course, for us and it may be like suffering a chronic disease thus we must balance ourselves as "being happy" with an understanding that the reality is, it is going to be an ongoing battle for our own survival. Depression will undermine even the strongest of wills, need help to maintain or at least be reminded of a happy outlook and happiness that is prevailing within us. Counseling, psychotherapy, and the right combination of medication will play a crucial role in helping to keep us from sinking into that very dark place that is the essence of depression and unhappiness. Be patient, but don't look for miracles. It may be that we will need the help of professionals throughout our lives to maintain a generally even keel. If one could "will away" depression, there would be no need of doctors or drugs. What we can do is understand why we feel like we do, and explain to our counselors that we wish it were that easy, and that we appreciate our concern towards being happy persons. Shifting our thoughts enables us to the right path of our happiness and thinking in its direction of positivity can make us to lead a very happy life.

LEAVE WORRIES NOW
BE HAPPY ENJOY LIFE

CHAPTER 12

BRING BACK YOUR LIFE TO NORMAL

We need to remember that as we possibly as we can we should make it a point to eat a more balanced, and healthy diet even though we may very little money left with us. We have intake of lot of greens vegetables and with variety of fruit and nuts which are all super healthy food for us, and which are less expensive than meats, cheeses, and processed foods! Their nitrifying value will energize and elevate our body, and knowing this that we are treating ourselves will surely refresh our minds. If we look for rich food rich in vitamins and other useful ingredients which include nuts, soya beans and fatty fish we would get more nutrition value. We must cut back on the caffeine drinks, alcohol. We don't have to quit, but reducing the intake of them will help reduce anxiety and stress from time to time.Exercise is one of health sport that our body needs most. It may be yoga, cross training, or even a simple walking in the park. This helps keeping our body active and will also help to grow our outlook. If we make it hobby we would enjoy the most. Whether its art, photography, music focusing on something other than the worry factor it will give our mind some good atmosphere to breathe off and would generate a good behavior within us. The other refreshing factor is naturally our sleep. We need not be reminded of this. Our body is probably begging us for it when we are in the middle of hard times. We may be drawn to maintain good sleeping habits. Maintain a consistent sleep schedule, but allow yourself some leeway. If we sleep peacefully let our body get about 8 hours of sleep we get the best results.

If you're just starting to have those thoughts, speak to your physician or your therapist. They may prescribe something to help steer you back to the center, emotionally. It may be the act of talking about it is therapeutic enough, but don't assume that. Leave that call to the professionals. Having goals which are set again and again after each one is achieved will give you a mindset or target to strive for which leads to success, with success becomes natural positive attitude. With all costiveness, goals and success builds a higher potential and belief within yourself. Setting realistic goals that you know you can achieve by staying positive is a great beginning to success. Your attitude around your friends, family and public people really tells them who you are, being positive instead of negative makes an excellent first impression on anybody. Positive means to be absolute, clear-cut, definite, forward-looking and expressively firm with a decision. Having a positive attitude toward something means you are willing to commit and do the work without complaint, which leads to goals. You realize that what appears negative today will change tomorrow. Nothing stays the same. Whether you are positive or negative, the situation does not change. So, we mind as well be positive. As with any habit, the habit of remaining positive in all situations takes practice and a commitment to yourself to take control. But start small, start paying attention to your emotions, start by wanting to change. Don't hold onto anything that bothers your mind. It can only hurt your health and it won't help your problems at all. The people that live the longest in this world do not hold grudges or hold onto negative feelings. Visualize your worries on a large chalkboard in your mind. Watch yourself take a big eraser and erase the problems. Every time the thoughts come back into your head, see yourself with the eraser again. Therefore do not worry about tomorrow, for tomorrow will worry about itself.

Each day has enough trouble of its own. Do not anticipate trouble, or worry about what may never happen. Keep in the sunlight. Imagine every day to be the last of a life surrounded with hopes, cares, anger and fear. The hours that come unexpectedly will be much the more grateful. The mind that is anxious about future events is miserable. Present fears are less than horrible imaginings. Let us be of good cheer, remembering that the misfortunes hardest to bear are those that never happen, focus on the positive aspects of their lives, rather than on the negative setbacks. "Feeling confident affects the way we perceive our situations and how we decide to manage them. Don't waste your life in doubts and fears: spend yourself on the work before you, well assured that the right performance of this hour's duties will be the best preparation for the hours or ages that follow it. It is not work that kills men, it is worry. Work is healthy; you can hardly put more on a man than he can bear. But worry is rust upon the blade. It is not movement that destroys the machinery, but friction. Never let life's hardships disturb you ... no one can avoid problems, not even saints or sages. As with any habit, the habit of remaining positive in all situations takes practice and a commitment to yourself to take control. Life is what you make it, so make it a happy one!! Don't worry on things that may not happen, life is too short to worry to0 much. Smile and be happy.

LEAVE WORRIES NOW
BE HAPPY ENJOY LIFE

HAVE HAPPINESSAND GOOD LIVING

Annalise sweet good and happy living and stop worrying over petty matters. Generate sweet living and generate good thoughts. Don't wait around or expect others to create happiness that is entirely yours to make. Whatever your goal is, do whatever you have to do to get it, always keep yourself to be a happy person. Why worry about the future. Just imagine as to what if we just acted like everything was easy and there was nothing very serious about it to come in future. Worry often gives a small thing a big shadow and its surrounding do frightened with more scary things with the result we do not tend to have a happy life or a sweet and happing living. Make yourself aware of what's possible in this world.

Worrying will carry tomorrow's load with today's strength. Worry will not empty tomorrow of its sorrows, but it tends to empty today of its power and strength. Worries make you to move into tomorrow ahead of time. Half the worry in the world is caused by people trying to make decisions before they have sufficient knowledge on which to base a decision. Their negative thoughts pressurise them to be away from the positivity in their lives as they fail and do not analysis on positive and they fail to lead a happy life or sweet life.

Concentrate on today's happening

Why worry about tomorrow. Concentrate on today happening as for tomorrow will worry about itself.

Each day has its own worries and troubles. Always think that you are a happy man. If there is not any solution to the some problem then do not waste time worrying about it. And if there is a solution to the problem then why waste time worrying about it. Act fast be happy generate positive happiness worries will automatically vanish in the air and you are sure to lead a sweet life and happy life.

The first step to good and happiness is by way of creating good and happy thoughts in your minds.

Focus your imagination and make efforts on becoming new positive person. Create happiness in you. Divert your mind to good thoughts. It is much easier to bring about change if you just put your mind to it and change your thoughts into a much more positive direction. We know that it is difficult for us to control things that happen in our lives, but we can, with some effort, control what we think or do in our lives. Positive thoughts will make our imagination livelier and we would be able to lead our lives happily without many worries.

The second good step is to have the company of good and positive living friends.

Appreciate the people in your life who have stood by you through thick and thin. Count their support and analyses the happiness in them which will help you to lead a much happier life. Good friends help each other in the days of crises and through both the good and bad times. Keep yourself busy and surround yourself with good friends, who always think positive. Feel positive about them and feel lucky to have them in your company. Share positive thoughts with them. Tell them to be happy and to lead a sweet good and happy life.

The third step is to focus your imagination on happy things in life by giving a good smile.

The easiest way is feeling happy. Many theories have revealed that happiness can lift one's mood and can divert your mind to sweet living. We may also share positivity with others by flashing them with a brilliant and good smile. Positive and sweet talks are the rewards of good and happy thoughts it generates more happiness. Dejection, disappointments and depression, however, have consequences that could ruin our health, and life. We must divert their minds to focus to the imagination of good and happy life. If something bad or good is to happen it is sure to happen, whether we are sad or unhappy or depressed. Let us put our energy into today and stop worrying about the future and past. We should not foresee trouble, or worry about what may never happen as past is dead and gone forever and future is uncertain and yet to come. Be your unabashed self in all the best ways that you can.

The basic facts we should know about happiness.

The basic techniques to analyze happiness and how to break the unhappy habits before it breaks us. These are the simple ways where we can concentrate and get rid of unhappy thoughts. Annalise unhappiness to see and get the reasons and facts as to why we worry. To avoid reoccurrence of worries, concentrate on prayers as prayers are the best source of remedies of the prevailing worries. The more you pray, the less you'll panic. The more you worship, the less you worry. There is nothing that wastes the body like worry, and anyone who has any faith in God should need not to worry about anything whatsoever is to happen in future. This will ease our way to a sweet good and happy living.

What do we think about happy thoughts?

The feeling of happiness is within us.

It is said that sweet good and happy living is purely our own matter and it has nothing to do with our external circumstances. There is something very special within us which keeps us happy and there is something very unpleasant within us which keeps unhappy. Yes quite true it is the positiveness within us that make and creates happiness within us. Happy living through positivity is nothing more than that of living a normal life free from undue pressures, problems and tensions. If we want to live a happy life then we need to get rid of the negativity and we must try to avoid all the unpleasant things within us which makes us unhappy.

Negative approach always complicates the problems and increases unhappiness.

Most of us do the fatal mistake of looking outwards for happiness rather than looking inwards. Be happy, be strong, be bold and be courageous every day. Even if we are having a bad day, think of some good things that may come our way, either later that day, tomorrow, next week, month, or next moment.

Simply making castles in the air won't solve our problems.

When everything seems to be beyond our control, it's almost too easy for us to slip into the grasp of unhappiness. To avoid unhappiness we must strive to abolish this sort of thinking through the power of thinking positively. We ought to know the basic fundamental of analyzing happiness.

Worries and unhappiness create unnecessary thoughts and these are caused by people going in for unwanted decisions, fore hand not even knowing as to when a good decision is made and not even having sufficient knowledge about it. We must first study and after carefully weighing all the facts than only come to a powerful decision. Simply making castles in the air won't solve our problems but add more to our vows and unhappiness which may even lead us to unhappy life. Anxiety and worry can go hand in hand. When anxiety grabs the mind, it is self-perpetuating. Your mind gets clogged with numerous buts and ifs. Do not worry about your life.

Negativity and worries are repetitive thoughts

Negativity and worries are repetitive thoughts associated with feelings of anxiety in anticipation of some negative future event. Worries and anxious feelings lead to disasters and make our lives unhappy. If we know that our circumstances are beyond our control or power we need to change them or revise them to our liking. We must try to put a stop-less order on our worries. We must be careful and we need not permit little things which become insects of our lives to ruin our happiness. Co-operate with the inevitable. Decide just how much anxiety a thing may be worth and refuse to give in anymore. All the happiness is not given in one go it comes slowly and slowly. We must pay special attention to remain happy and be happy. Keep ourselves happy, treat our worried thoughts as valuable signals to a sweet living good and happy living.

The utmost cause of unhappiness is your state of depression. Unhappiness is not there to motivate information gathering or problem-solving. In fact it is depression that constructs the future of unhappiness.

Depression is inertia. That's the thing about depression: depression is so insidious, and it compounds daily, and it's impossible to ever see the end of it.

Keep yourself happy

Depressed people think they know themselves, but maybe they only know depression. There are no hopeless than this to get depressed create unhappiness in our minds and become unhappy all the time. Our attitude towards suffering and depression becomes very important because it can affect how we cope with suffering when it arises. Depression is nourished by a lifetime of grieved and unforgiven causes. Another factor to remain unhappy is worrying about unwanted and useless things. Worry is a misuse of the imagination. To keep yourself happy, treat your worried thoughts as most unwanted assets. These are the fundamental facts you should be familiar about worries. A huge factor to stay happy is to cater your worries around, an important relationship in your life and pay special attention sustaining positive relationships. Make your mind firm and do come to a positive decision and not allow the worries to un-ease the power your mind and soul that can cause unhappiness in you.

We must free ourselves from fruitless worry.

Once a decision is carefully reached we should get busy carrying out our decisions and should not bother about all the anxieties that are about to come. When we, or any of our colleagues or associates, are about to worry about a problem, we must write it out and think of the following questions: Instead of worrying about what people say, why not spend time trying to accomplish something they may admire. What if we just acted like everything was easy?

How would your life be different if we stopped worrying about things we can't control and started focusing on the things we can? Let today be the day. We must free ourselves from fruitless worry, seize the day and take effective action on things we can change thus we would see that our lives changes for the betterment and we are on the right path of a sweet, good and happy living.

LEAVE WORRIES NOW BE HAPPY ENJOY LIFE

CHAPTER 14

GET MORE HAPPINESS

If you are interested in getting more success and happiness within you, focus on all the ways as if you have already attained success. You need to focus on the thing and create a happy live within you. If you want love and affection, focus on all the people and the abundance of love that you have to give to them. If we want to have greater health, focus on all the ways that we are healthy, thus creating and delivering a good life within you. You need to admit that there are problems that you cannot change. But you can change the way of your thinking if you identify the main reason of the problem. And if you acknowledge the facts, that you have been negative or inactive in finding a solution to the problem, probably this will make it easier for you to become positive thus creating a new lease of life within you. It will make your life easier to lead a good and sweet life.

You must try to make goals

You must try to make goals. Making goals can give you a more positive outlook on life. People often tend to get bored with life and get the feeling that they are stuck to negative things which the result they often get the feeling of being depressed. Setting a direction for yourself and a goal would surely help you to move forward.

Mental attitude that can bring you peace and happiness

If you expecting to succeed, and are not afraid of failure, you have the best chance of staying positive and can create a very positive life within you. When you, or any of your associates, are tempted to worry about a problem, write out the solution and a definite answer to it. This helps a positive feeling to generate within you making you very positive to have a good living. Another thing you need to understand is that there are several ways to cultivate a mental attitude that can bring you peace and happiness and can carnage a good life within you. More of it if you fill your mind with thoughts of peace, courage, health, and hope, your life will be easy to live. You would get a happy feeling of life and mind if you let yourself to forget your own unhappiness, by trying to create a little happiness for others. You are best to yourself and to others.

The first step is to write down your worries

The first step is to write down your worries, which will help you make sense of them, and then decide on one small step you can take towards a solution. But to be very true no man in this world is free of obstacles or difficulties. Don't make worry your habit. Break this habit and stop all the negative and panic thoughts provoking your mind all the time. If you can't change the past, but you must not ruin the present by worrying about the future. Joy is what happens to us when we allow ourselves to recognize how good things really are. When we feel worried and depressed, we need to consciously form a smile on our faces and act upbeat until the happy feeling becomes genuine reality.

Happiness is what is needed most.

What makes to lead a happy life is not to get trapped into unnecessary unwanted worries and negative thoughts.

Don't create the feeling of depression and anger. Feelings of depression and hopelessness and or anger are even tougher to cope with on a consistent basis. When you are worried, you not only hurt yourself, but the limited support systems that are still holding on your mind but making you to get more and more worried and nothing is achieved in terms of success except the re-carnation of worries and worries thus leading you to be unhappy and worried all the time. Your actions breed confidence and courage. If you want to conquer fear, anger and worry do not sit ideal and just think about it. Let our deep worrying become advance thinking and planning. If you look into your own mind and heart, and you find nothing wrong there, what is there to worry about? Practically nothing what is there to fear about and again nothing? So why worry unnecessarily and make your present and future dark. Neglect all those which make your life unhappy.

Why being a negative person?

Why being a negative person and what do you get out of it being a depression dejected and sad man.? Why not turn your thoughts to be a positive person simply it is a question of tilting your mind towards a positive side of thing. See both the aspects of a situation and ways the pros and cons of both the sides and try to abolish the negativity in you. Be positive strong and you will remain happy for ever. We all have different roles that we play in the lives of people we love and care about. Our actions and how well we play our part has a direct influence on their life, so we better get in there and give our best performance. Tell them with how much you care in the capacity that you're in. At the end of the day, money is just a means to an end. Nothing more.

If you're grinding and struggling to make ends meet and buried under piles of debt, that's pretty stressful. Once you have your basic needs met though, more money only makes you happier up to a certain point. Money cannot buy you happiness. You need to generate it yourself. Someone will always be better than you at something, but it does not matter. Be inspired by them, using it to push yourself further, and nothing more. If they can do it, why cannot you?

Are you are interested in getting more happiness?.

If you are interested in getting more happiness focus on all the ways as if you have already attained success. You need to focus on the thing and create a live within you. If you want love and affection, focus on all the people and the abundance of love that you have to give to them.

Worrisome thoughts reproduce faster.

Worrisome thoughts reproduce faster so one of the most powerful ways to stop the spiral of worry is simply to disclose the worry to a friend. Practice happy gratitude daily. Take three minutes at the end of your day to chill and write down a small list of the things that can make you smile, laugh, or that you're glad are a part of your life. There's something to be grateful about, especially when you look down at that list and realize that a lot of people have it worse off than you do and could use a few of those things. Simply being an optimist will not solve all your problems, but what's the alternative is to keep your mind and heart cool and always have happy and positive feeling and think that life is to live happily. There isn't much sense in being anything else.

If you're constantly filling your head with negative thoughts, odds are they'll lead you straight towards negative actions, self-doubt and increase the general happiness of life isn't a cool place to live at all. Think of each setback as a challenge to see the positive, spin the situation back around, making it better than it was before and start living in a good and sweet manner.

What do we get out of unhappiness?

We may feel largely uncomfortable, when worries attack our thoughts and mind. While we are consuming more worries we are far too busy to do anything else to fix the real problem and would rather find it hard to get into a smart solution. Thus resulting in a fact that you spend your evenings worrying only without even bothering to find some time to know its cause We get nothing out of worrying except only to think and cry and become unhappy. We do not get anything out of unhappiness. Another thing is that we may feel largely uncomfortable, when worries attack our thoughts and mind which makes worrying about a situation an easier option to get depressed and diffused. While we are consuming more worries we are far too busy to do anything else to fix the real problem and would rather find it hard to get into a smart solution. Thus resulting in a fact that we spend our evenings worrying only without even bothering to find some time to search a sweet happiness within us. Negative thought which are provoking our mind, about the uncertainties and the negativities, as to what will happen tomorrow creates unnecessary worries and worries are repetitive thoughts associated with feelings of anxiety in anticipation of some negative future event which may end in a failure.

Whether the worries are about financial crisis, family problems, work, health or any topic of concern, the anxious feelings and negative thoughts produced are always distinctly unpleasant thus making us unhappy all the time. We get nothing being a negative and unhappy man. We must not forget that if we tend to worry they will never rob tomorrow of its sorrows, but will only deny today of its meaning happiness and joys. Negative thoughts only produce worries and worrying is actually a form of superstition and creates false images in our mind and that is the main reason and cause which makes and leads us to this point of imagination. A human being can survive almost anything, as long as he or she sees the end in sight, starts analyzing his positive thoughts and starts analyzing his unhappiness.

We need to fore see the coming trouble first.

We must not forgot that if something bad or good is to happen it is sure to happen, whether we worry or not. Let us put our energy into today and stop worrying about the future and past. We should not foresee trouble, or worry about what may never happen as past is dead and gone forever and future is uncertain and yet to come. Positive thinking our brave attitude and our courage will ward off everything and bring happiness in our lives. The basic facts we should know about worry. The basic techniques to analyze worry and how to break the worry habit before it breaks us. These are the simple ways where we can concentrate and get rid of worries prevailing in our thoughts, remove all the negativity in our live and start living a positive good and happy life.

Think of good and positive ways of Happy Living.

Annalise positive ways of happy living and get to see the reasons and facts of worry. To avoid reoccurrence of worries, concentrate on prayers as prayers are the best source of remedies of the prevailing worries. Think good ways of living and starting praying. The more you pray, the less you'll panic. The more you worship, the less you worry. There is nothing that wastes the body like worry, and anyone who has any faith in God should need not to worry about anything whatsoever is to happen in future. Positive thinking is the creation of good imagination and good imagination is the creation of sweet and happy living.

Happiness comes with Positive living and sweet thoughts

If you know that the circumstance is beyond your control or power change than revise it to your liking. Just try to put a stop-less order on your worries. Don't permit little things which become insects of life to ruin your happiness. Co-operate with the inevitable. Decide just how much anxiety a thing may be worth and refuse to give in anymore.

All the happiness is not given in one go it comes slowly and slowly with positive thinking.

Have worry under your control. If your worries center around, pay special attention to remain positive and be happy. Keep yourself happy, treat your worried thoughts as valuable signals. How to keep from worrying about criticism? Simply unjust criticism and think positively and do often discard a bad compliment. It often means that you have aroused jealousy and envy. Let's keep a record of the fool things we have done and stop criticizing ourselves.

Cause of unhappiness is Negative way of living life

The utmost cause of worry is our negative thinking as it leads us to the state of depression. Living will change for the better-If You Think Positive. Our negative thinking and attitude towards suffering and depression becomes very important because it can affect how we cope with suffering when it arises. Depression is nourished by a lifetime of un-grieved and unforgiven causes. Times will change for the better when you change. Worry is a misuse of the imagination. Worry is most often a prideful way of thinking that you have more control over life and its circumstances than you actually do. Positive Thinking leads your way to good and happiness. An art of Good and Happy Living.

Neglect worries keep yourself happy.

Neglect worries keep yourself happy, treat your worried thoughts as valuable signals. These are the fundamental facts you should be familiar about worries. A huge factor to stay happy is to cater your worries around, an important relationship in your life and pay special attention sustaining positive relationships. Worries are there to motivate information gathering and problem-solving. Make your mind firm and do come to a positive decision as come what we will not allow the worries to entire our mind and soul.

What if we just acted like everything was easy?

Once a decision is carefully reached we should get busy carrying out our decisions and should not bother about all the anxieties that are about to come. When we, or any of our colleagues or associates, are about to worry about a problem, we must write it out and think positively of the questions. Instead of worrying about what people say of you, why not spend time trying to accomplish something they will admire.

What if we just acted like everything was easy? How would your life be different if you stopped worrying about things we can't control and started focusing on the things we can? Let today be the day. Free yourself from fruitless worry, seize the day and take effective action on things you can change. We would change ourselves for the betterment if we start thinking in positive terms. Positive thinking is what is required of us and simply worrying about the future things or as to what will happen in the next moment will certainly deprive us of good and happy living that we are about gather or get in the next hour.

Another cause of getting worried or unhappy is the attachment

Attachment brings worry. If you have a problem and you come up with the answer, you stop worrying immediately. Our minds can be dishonest, persuading us that we are worrying about something, when our deepest fear is entirely different. No-one likes to admit that they've chosen to worry. The first step is to write down your worries, which will help you make sense of them, and then decide on one small step you can take towards a solution. But to be very true no man in this world is free of obstacles or difficulties. Don't make worry your habit. Break this habit and stop all the negative and panic thoughts provoking your mind all the time if you want to remain a happy person and lead a happy good and sweet life. Feelings of depression and angry are even tougher to cope with on a consistent basis. When you are worried, you not only hurt yourself, but the limited support systems that are still holding on your mind making you to get more and more worried and nothing is achieved in terms of success except the re-carnation of worries and worries.

Joy is what happens to us when we allow ourselves to recognize how good things really are.

Practically nothing what is there to fear about?

So why worry unnecessarily and make your present and future dark. Why being a negative person and what do you get out of it being a depression dejected and sad man.? Why not turn your thoughts to be a positive person simply it is a question of tilting your mind towards a positive side of thing. See both the aspects of a situation and ways the pros and cons of both the sides and try to abolish the negativity in you. You will surely be a happy man.

Think of the best the best is sure to happen

Think of the best the best is sure to happen and if you think of the worst the worst will come. Better come forward wake up and think positive first. Positive persons always succeed in life whatever be the circumstances and the negative often dig a death trap for themselves. So why be a negative person why you have all the qualities of being a positive man. Surround yourself with friends and people that are better than you in areas that you want to improve in.

LEAVE WORRIES NOW
BE HAPPY ENJOY LIFE

CHAPTER 15

BE STRONG IT WILL GENERATE HAPPINESS

If you are interested in getting more happiness, focus on all the ways as if you have already attained success. You need to focus on the thing and create a live within you. Positive thinking will generate happiness in you. Our actions positive thinking breed confidence and courage in us. If we want to conquer fear, anger and worry we should sit ideal and just think about it. Let our deep worrying do some advance thinking and planning. If we look into our own mind and heart, and we will find nothing wrong there, what is there to worry about and generate unhappiness in us?

Is there anything to be unhappy about?

Practically nothing what is there to be unhappy about? So why worry unnecessarily and make our present and future dark. Discard negative thought think positive and be happy. Positive thinking is the key to all problems and worries. Solve all your problems and get rid of all unnecessary worries by simply thinking in a positive manner. What is there to worry about? Think positive, be positive and have confidence in you. You will create great happiness within yourself. You need to admit that there are problems that you cannot change. But you can change the way of your thinking if you identify the main reason of the problem. And if you acknowledge the facts, that you have been negative or inactive in finding a solution to the problem, probably this will make it easier for you to become positive thus creating a new lease of life within you.

You must try to make goals.

Making goals can give you a more positive outlook on life. People often tend to get bored with life and get the feeling that they are stuck to negative things which the result they often get the feeling of being depressed. Setting a direction for yourself and a goal would surely help you to move forward. If you expecting to succeed, and are not afraid of failure, you have the best chance of staying positive and can create a very positive life within you. When you, or any of your associates, are tempted to worry about a problem, write out the solution and a definite answer to it. This helps a positive feeling to generate within you.

There are several ways to cultivate a mental attitude.

Another thing you need to understand is that there are several ways to cultivate a mental attitude that can bring you peace and happiness and can carnage a good life within you. More of it if you fill your mind with thoughts of peace, courage, health, and hope, your life will be easy to live. You would get a happy feeling of life and mind if you let yourself to forget your own unhappiness, by trying to create a little happiness for others. You are best to yourself. The perfect way to conquer worry is the Prayer of God. To keep yourself from worrying about criticism, do not even try to get mixed with your enemies, because if you do you will hurt yourself far more than we hurting them. Instead of worrying about ingratitude, let's expect it. Let's remember that the only way to find happiness is not to expect gratitude, but to give for the joy of giving. Let us build a happy life within us generate peace and a healthy atmosphere around us.

Let us build a happy life within us

This will help us to lead a peaceful happy and prosperous life and we would find ourselves to be happier than before. You should do things in the order of their importance. You need to clear your desk of all papers except those relating to the immediate problem at hand. When you face a problem, solve it then and there, if you have the facts to make a decision. Make a decision fast and do not linger on. Learn to organize, deputize, and supervise and straight away come to decision. Simply postponing it would spoil your good thoughts and there is every likelihood your mind may get into negative activities and start thinking in negative manner. Therefore write down a list of things that make you excited, however big, small, likely or unlikely. Then work to make them occur more often. Look for moments of joy and savor them. Recognize your good happening every day.

Eat well do plenty of exercise and do not skip meals.

It is a known fact that physical exercise is known to stimulate our veins and get to strengthen our minds that lift depression and anxiety so we need to walk, swim, run or whatever we like doing best. Those who create or those who do well on the worst scenario, give themselves worry and stress, tend to be devastated. If we cannot get some sunshine, we can always lighten up our rooms with brighter lights. We can have lunch outside the office. Take frequent walks instead of driving our cars over short distances. No man is indispensable. First of all our circle of friends is always there to give us some moral support. Spending time and engaging ourselves in worthwhile activities could give us a very enjoyable and satisfying feeling. Nothing feels better than having group support.

Good friends are quite important and their company generally lightened up our spirits. To get to know and to find such friends we simply have to be friendly with ourselves, and then the friendships will naturally follow us.

We need to understand the power of touch and support and we have not to underestimate it strength and support. Don't we feel so good when someone pats us on our back and gives us some words of encouragement during your most challenging times and difficult times? Just hug or embrace someone someday you will see that you have almost changed his life. Get intimate with him and try to establish close ties with his family and friends. The love and care expressed by you will tremendously boost him and well as your immune system and fury of worry will be diminished for all.

In our lives storms may come and go.

In our lives storms may come and go. in the form of reversals, but if we have the power and foundation of inner fulfillment and if we deal with it with a very clear practical mind these storms will not kill us or will not disrupt us. There could be numberless reasons for which we keep on worrying. We may be worried about our health, wealth, loved ones, friends, the happening of yesterday and the follow happenings of tomorrow. The environment or the world politics, but these can be dealt with firm mind and fearless worry if we generate within ourselves the power of enlightenment within ourselves. There's no sense in worrying about the negatives if these negatives cannot be changed. If we waste energy and happiness on the things we can't change, we'll only make ourselves more frustrated and come to the stage of depression dejection and disappointments.

Negativity is a habit.

Negativity is a habit and we often don't realize we're doing ourselves down. Under each negative thought that we have written, we can spot an alternative way of looking at it, that isn't so negative. Take your mind to positivity and mold and drive your thoughts to the positivity. There's a world of difference between expecting failure or rejection so as not to be disappointed when it occurs and recognizing it as a possibility of being positive. It's sensible to look at a situation from all angles and to have a back-up plan to fall back on if need be. People who do this will not see failure as another step on the road to eventual success; but by expecting and envisioning success, there's less likely to be a failure. Let us find some ways of removing negative thoughts and discouraging our worries to be born.

Let us all generate and create happiness within us

Let us all generate and create happiness within us by removing all negative thoughts negative feeling and unwanted desires that make our mind greedy and spoil the charm of our sweet good and happy living. Remember three aspects - naturalness, simplicity and belongingness. Just open up your heart and be natural. Next is living a simple life. Living with the confidence will get whatever is needed, that is simplicity. Right or wrong, we are what we are. We need to tone our life accordingly and if we live like this naturally, then there will not be any fear. There will be no doubts or blocks in life. This is the important mantra of Art of Sweet Living. Another important thing is that if we cannot get some good sunshine, we can always lighten up our thoughts with brighter lights of happy living. We can have ample of lunch of positive thinking. To avoid negative thoughts we need to take frequent walks.

No man is indispensable and no man is not capable of positive thinking. Let us make ourselves happy and life become a sweet living.

Happiness is a state of mind.

We know the saying, that "Happiness is a state of mind". And state of mind is what we think and what we do or act in a peaceful manner without being getting worried or depressed. If you are interested in getting more happiness, to get it through positive thinking. All we need to do is to focus on all the directions on positive thinking and happy living as if we have already attained success. We need to focus on the thing and create a life within us. If we want love and affection, entertain people and give them the abundance of love.

If we want to have greater health, pay attention on all the ways that make us healthy, thus creating and delivering a good life within us by thinking in positive ways. We need to understand and admit that there are problems that we cannot change. But we can change the ways of our thinking and if we identify the main reason of the problem we can remove all the obstacles coming in our way of leading a sweet and happy life. And if we acknowledge the fact, that we have been negative or inactive in finding a solution to the problem, this will make it easier for us to become positive thus creating a new lease of life within us.

Positive thinking will surely make us happy.

Another thing to understand is that we must try to make our goals. Making goals can give us a more positive outlook on life.

People often tend to get bored with life and get the feeling that they are stuck to negative things with the result they often get the feeling of being depressed dejected and monotonous and become unhappy in life. Setting a direction and a goal for ourselves, would surely help us to move forward. If we are expecting to succeed, and are not afraid of failure, we stand the best chance of staying positive and thus can create a very positive life within us.

Mental attitude that can bring you peace and happiness.

Another thing you need to understand is that there are several ways to cultivate a mental attitude that can bring you peace and happiness and can carnage a good life within you. More of it if you fill your mind with thoughts of peace, courage, health, and hope, your life will be easy to live. If you think in positive terms you would get a happy feeling of life and mind you if you let yourself to forget your own unhappiness, by trying to create a little happiness for others you are sure to get happiness in your live. You are best to yourself. The perfect way to conquer worry is the Prayer of God. You should do things in the order of their importance.

Learn to think in positive terms.

When you face a problem, solve it then and there, by thinking positively and if you have the facts of making a decision, make a decision fast and do not linger on. Learn to think in positive terms organize the things, deputise, and supervise straight away by coming to decision. To keep yourself from worrying about criticism, do not even try to get mixed with your enemies, because if you do you will hurt yourself far more than we hurting them.

You will fall prey to negative thinking and this in turn will lead you unhappiness in life. Simply postponing it would spoil your good thoughts and there is every likelihood your mind may get into negative activities and start thinking in negative manner. Therefore think positive, write down a list of things that make you positive, however big, small, likely or unlikely. Then work to make them occur more often. Look for moments of joy and savor them. Recognise your good happening every day. Be positive think positive and be happy.

Happiness is your own choice and decision

You may also feel that life has become terrible for you to live and you are carrying no hope that someone would be there to rescue you. Happiness is your own choice and decision. Each of us can be as happy as we make up our minds to be. We can, if we want, fill up our days with positive attitude chatter and laughter. To be happy, we need to concentrate only on happy thoughts. Our friends are always there to give us some moral support. Spending time and engaging ourselves in worthwhile positive activities could give us a very enjoyable and satisfying feeling. Nothing feels better than having group support and talking in terms of positive thinking. Good friends are quite important and their company generally lightened up our spirits. This makes us to think in positive manner and to get to know such friends we simply have to be friendly with ourselves, and then the friendships will naturally follow us and make our lives happy.

Only way to find happiness is not to expect gratitude.

Let us remember that the only way to find happiness is not to expect gratitude, but to give for the joy of giving.

Let us build a happy life within us generate peace and a healthy atmosphere around us. This will help us to lead a peaceful happy and prosperous life and we would find ourselves to be happier than before. We need to understand the power of positive thinking and its support and we have not to underestimate it strength and support. Don't we feel so good when someone pats us on our back and gives us some words of encouragement during your most challenging times and difficult times and advises us to remain positive and think positive just hug or embrace someone with positive attitude someday? We will see that we have almost changed our life.

The ghosts of the past have to be exorcised. We may be working in any field, the key to success is our outlook. Sometimes we may think that no road is left for us from where we can achieve the happiness of life. One need not to forget that we need to eat well do plenty of exercise and do not skip meals. It is a known fact that physical exercise is known to stimulate our veins and get to strengthen our minds that lift depression and anxiety, so we need to walk, swim, run or whatever we like doing best above all we must move ahead in direction where our mind can generate electricity to think in positive directly and bring immense happiness to us

Difficulties and storms may come and go.

In our lives difficulties and storms may come and go in the form of reversals, but if we have the power of positive thinking and foundation of inner fulfillment we would be able to deal with it with a very clear practical mind and with this positive thinking these storms will not kill us nor will disrupt us. There could be numberless reasons for which we keep on worrying.

We may be worried about our health, wealth, loved ones, friends, the happening of yesterday and the follow happenings of tomorrow, the environment or the world politics, but these can be dealt with firm mind and fearless worry if we generate within ourselves the power of positive thinking within ourselves and try to be happy all the time.

The best thing about happiness is that we get it is free.

We don't have to pay or we do not have to open any account to be happy. We don't have to pay monthly rent for it either. WE just have to change our perspective, our views on what we are seeing and feeling. Happiness is not something which is quite readymade. It comes from our own actions and deeds.

Angriness and happiness don't mix.

We must dig out the angriness in us, and see that the happiness has shown and seeded a place to grow its roots. The ultimate goal of life should be to get happiness and not get involved into unnecessary worries falling in the death trap of defeats and failures. The essence of life is not in the great victories and grand failures, but in the simple joys. The purpose of our lives is to be happy.

If you want to be happy, be positive first practice meditation.

Laugh when you can, apologize when you should, and let go of what you can't change. Think positive and just visualize that what is stored in destiny would not be negative. If you want to be happy, be positive first practice meditation. If you want, others to be happy practice compassion. Whoever is happy will make others happy, too.

Happiness doesn't depend on any superficial conditions.

Let us be very sure and let us keep in mind that happiness doesn't depend on any superficial conditions, it is governed by our mental attitude only. Our greatest gift to others is to be happy and to radiate our happiness to the entire world. Happiness is a guide to direction, not a place to hide. As a happy person, we radiate happiness to the world. We need to visualise our light radiating throughout the world, passing from person to person until it encircles the globe. Resolve to keep happy, and you shall form an invincible host against difficulties.

The path to happiness is forgiveness.

The positive persons often dance to the happy tunes of their lives. The path to happiness is forgiveness of everyone and gratitude for everything. Happiness fills our heart each day and our whole life through with clean thoughts. Any day would be a wonderful day if we do not to take life so seriously. Happiness is not about being a winner it is about being gentle with life being gentle within us. Happiness blooms in the presence of self-respect and the absence of ego. Love yourself. Love everyone around you. Love everyone in the whole world. When you're feeling depressed or anxious, close your eyes and try to visualize a guided positive imaginary thing. First breathe deeply and relax. How important it is to consistently reach for positive, uplifting, inspirational thoughts. Thought that promote aliveness and abundance. Thoughts that make you feel good. Imagine that you are already a positive person and you love life.

Happiness can only be achieved if you have a positive mind.

The only thing between us and our desire, to be happy, is one single fact: we are not happy because we often fall into the death trap of depression and wholly because of our negative thoughts. Absence of positive thinking, has eluded us of our great happiness and left us far behind. This very little known fact has kept many of us from reaching our goal of happiness. Throw away all your negative thoughts and worries, concentrate on the goals to be achieved, on the ray of happiness in you and make sure that you are not falling again into the path of negativity. Happiness is a state of mind only and not the thoughts of negatives, and it quite true that happiness can only be achieved if you have a positive mind and a clear attitude of being a positive person. Happiness and positivity go hand in hand. If you are positive you are a happy person and if you possess negativity you would land yourself to be a very negative person thus ruining your life for what of nothing with the result you become an unhappy person and you remain aloof from leading a sweet good and happy living.

LEAVE WORRIES NOW
BE HAPPY ENJOY LIFE

CHAPTER 16

HAVE SWEET LIFE

We need to remember that as possibly as we can we should make it a point to eat a more balanced, and healthy diet even though we may very little money left with us. We have to take lot of greens vegetables and with variety of fruit and nuts which are all super healthy food for us, and which are more or less expensive than meats, cheeses, and processed foods. Their nitrifying value will energize and elevate our body, and knowing this that we are treating ourselves will surely refresh our minds and make us to lead a happy life. If we look for rich food rich in vitamins and other useful ingredients which include nuts, soya beans and fatty fish we would get more nutrition value. We must cut back on the caffeine drinks, alcohol. We don't have to quit, but reducing the intake of them will help reduce anxiety and stress from time to time thus making us to have more comforts leading to a happy and sweet life.

A positive person anticipates happiness, health and success.

We need to change our attitude from negative thinking to positive thinking and converge ourselves from negativity to positivity. Positive thinking is a mental and emotional attitude that focuses on the bright side of life and expects positive results.

A positive person anticipates happiness, health and success, and believes he or she can overcome any obstacle and difficulty. No matter how difficult the situation may appear. We should recognize the beautiful lessons waiting to be discovered. Sometimes lessons may prove to be expensive and costly, but every problem is a learning experience in disguise. We need to be conscious of our thoughts, especially, when life just is not going our way. The moment we see that we are diving into frustration, agony, sorrow or low self –esteem we must shift our thoughts, by thinking about something completely different and unrelated and always try to bring happiness in our lives irrespective of all the problems that we have been facing and are aware of it.

UNHAPPY LIVING IS MISERABLE

We affect, and are affected by the people we meet, in one way or another. This happens instinctively and on a subconscious level, through words, thoughts and feelings, and through body language. Is it any wonder that we want to be around positive and happy people, and prefer to avoid negative ones? People are more disposed to help us, if we are positive and happy, and they dislike and avoid anyone broadcasting unhappiness. Negative thoughts, words and attitude, create negative and unhappy feelings, moods and behavior. When the mind is negative, poisons are released into the blood, which cause more unhappiness and negativity. This is the way to failure, frustration and disappointment and unhappiness comes gushing in our minds. Individuals with a pessimistic explanatory style often blame themselves when bad things happen, but fail to give themselves adequate credit for successful outcomes.

They also have a tendency to view negative events as expected and lasting. As you can imagine, blaming yourself for events outside of your control or viewing these unfortunate events as a persistent part of your life can have a detrimental impact on your state of mind. Positive thinkers are more apt to use an optimistic explanatory style, but the way in which people attribute events can also vary depending upon the exact situation. This will strangle the pattern of self-pity, mind-created imaginations, and negative downward stairs.

What makes us different from other mammals is our ability to control our thoughts.

What makes us different from other mammals is our ability to control our thoughts and think for ourselves positively and shift our negative thoughts to a positive angle. We may have made mistakes, but now we can accept it and continue, knowing that we will make a different decision in the future. If we understand this it can be appreciative for the experience. We cannot be both angry and grateful at the same time. We should start counting the blessings and miracles in our lives and if we start exploring for them and we would find more. It's quite true that we are alive and breathing! We have to realize how lucky we are with all the happiness in abundance in our lives. Our mind and body becomes dumb and mum when it comes to pressure, all it wants to do is take the easiest way out and to throw out of us our negative within us making us to forgo happiness and adopt unhappiness in life. While the terms happy living and positive psychology are sometimes used interchangeably, it is important to understand that they are not the same thing.

First, happy living is about looking at things from a positive point of view. Positive psychology certainly tends to focus on optimism, but it also notes that while there are many benefits to thinking positively, there are actually times when more realistic thinking is more advantageous. Feeling good about ourselves and showing self-confidence boosts our skills potential and capabilities in any areas of work and supports us to become happier a person. We need to shift our thoughts from being a negative person to more strong a positive man. Also keeping in mind that pushing things to the limit and going beyond what we think is possible for us to get to the next step of being a happy man. It becomes another key to achieving what we really want to do.

Smiling laughing is the best medicine to a sweet living.

Yes all these are the best medicine. Based on the same concept above about smiling, laughing burns calories, increases our adrenaline and boosts health. There are even groups of people that get together just to laugh together. They are not laughing at jokes, they are just laughing for good health.

As with smiling, we do not need to laugh at real things, we just need to do the physical laughing for all of the health benefits. Even small amounts of exercise make us feel better. Let us take a walk if we are feeling bluesy, angry or slipping into negative thinking. We would have had someone tell us to "look on the brighter side" of any situation or problem disturbing us.

Even if it may be relationships and we are finding it difficult to meet someone where we are actually interested in, we need not wait because it usually does not come to us by own, we must stand up to get help from any learned fellow to guide us to a sweet and happy living. One of the most important things while doing all is to be happy about what we are doing, thus we ought to have a successful goal setting our lifestyle with a positive attitude. At times we may suffer from chronic depression, though we know how good things look on to others life cannot be worse for us.

Most import thing is to be happy and feel happy.

Let's imagine how to deal when life leaves a great big steaming pile at our doorstep. Lest we need to remember that external factors can be dealt with by taking positive steps to repair or at least address the root of the problem as best as we can. Whatever may be the primary cause of the problem, that cause must be examined first? We may or may not be able to solve the problem, but at least knowing that we are taking positive steps can help us improve our outlook. It will not be easy, of course, for us and it may be like suffering a chronic disease thus we must balance ourselves as being happy with an understanding that the reality is, and is not going to be an ongoing battle for our own survival. Depression will undermine even the strongest of wills, need help to maintain or at least be reminded of a positive outlook. Counseling, psychotherapy, and the right combination of medication will play a crucial role in helping to keep us from sinking into that very dark place that is the essence of depression.

Shifting our thoughts enables us to the right path of our happiness and thinking in its direction of happiness can make us to lead a very happy life.

Exercise is one of health sport that our body needs most.

It may be yoga, cross training, or even a simple walking in the park. This helps keeping our body active and will also help to grow our outlook. If we make it hobby we would enjoy the most. Whether its art, photography, music focusing on something other than the worry factor it will give our mind some good atmosphere to breathe off and would generate a good behavior within us. The other refreshing factor is naturally our sleep. We need not be reminded of this. Our body is probably begging us for it when we are in the middle of hard times. We may be drawn to maintain good sleeping habits. Maintain a consistent sleep schedule, but allow yourself some leeway. If we sleep peacefully let our body get about good hours of sleep we get the best results this in turn will lean us to lead a happy and sweet living instead of disturbed life. If we are starting to have those unhappy thoughts, we need to speak to our physician or our therapist. They may prescribe something to help steer us back to the center, emotionally. It may be the act of talking about it is therapeutic enough, but don't assume that. Let us leave that call to the professionals. Having goals which are set again and again after each one is achieved will give us a mindset or target to strive for which leads to success, with success becomes natural happy attitude.

With all costiveness, goals and success build a higher potential and belief within ourselves. Setting realistic goals that we know we can achieve by staying positive is a great beginning to a happy living.

We need to realize that what appears negative today will change tomorrow.

Nothing stays the same. Whether we are happy or unhappy, the situation does not change. Our attitude around our friends, family and people really tells them as to who we are and also being happy instead of unhappy makes an excellent first impression on anybody. Happiness means to be absolute, clear-cut, definite, forward looking and expressively firm with a decision. Having a happy attitude toward something means we are willing to commit and do the work without complaint, which leads to goals of happiness and sweet living. If a problem is fixable, and if a situation is such that we can do something about it, then there is no need to worry. If it is not fixable, then there is no help in worrying. There is no benefit in worrying whatsoever. If we have a problem, the thing to do is to communicate: find out the information we need to get the full picture, so that the solution becomes apparent. If we are upset, we need to communicate and say how we feel. If we have done something wrong, again we need to communicate. The nature of this world is that we have to face birth, old age, disease and death. Everything is always changing. The biggest problem is that we want to control our environment to our own wish and will and in turn remain unhappy since we are not able to achieve it even after all the efforts are put in to lead a happy life.

We must not hold on to anything that bothers our mind.

 It can only hurt our health and it won't help our problems
at all. The people that live the longest in this world do not
hold grudges or hold onto negative feelings. We need to
visualize our worries on a large chalkboard in our mind.
Watch yourself take a big eraser and erase the problems.
Every time the thoughts come back into our head, we need
to see ourselves with the eraser again. Let us keep our slate
clean. Unnecessary worry does not empty tomorrow of its
sorrow, it empties today of its strength and tends to make
us unhappy all the time. Worrying does not empty
tomorrow of its sorrow, it empties today of its strength. If
we are worried about the future. Life is what we make it, so
make it a happy one. We need not worry on things that
may not happen, life is too short to worry too much. Smile
and be happy and start living a sweet and happy life.
Recent studies have shown that smiling can increase our
good health. We receive the same benefits whether we feel
like smiling or not. Smiling also benefits everyone that sees
it. Smiling at others makes them feel good too. So smile,
fake or not, it is good for us and good for our recipient. It is
the best medicine. Based on the same concept above about
smiling, laughing burns calories, increases our adrenaline
and boosts health. There are even groups of people that get
together just to laugh together. They are not laughing at
jokes, they are just laughing for good health. As with
smiling, we do not need to laugh at real things, we just need
to do the physical laughing for all of the health benefits.
Even small amounts of exercise make us feel better. All
this tips help us to maintain a good happy and sweet living.

LEAVE WORRIES NOW
BE HAPPY ENJOY LIFE

CHAPTER 17

FORGET NEGATIVITY

Thought which are provoking our mind, about the uncertainties and the negativities, as to what will happen tomorrow. The root causes of this negatives are the creation of worries in our minds. The fundamental thought provoking heart and mind are the worries that are growing rapidly within us. Worries are repetitive thoughts associated with feelings of anxiety in anticipation of some negative future event. Whether the worries are about financial crisis, family problems, work, health or any topic of concern, the anxious feelings produced and sustained by the imaginary thoughts which always distinctly appear to be unpleasant. Worrying will carry tomorrow's load with today's strength. Worry will not empty tomorrow of its sorrows, it empties today of its power and strength. Worries make you to move into tomorrow ahead of time. Half the worry in the world is caused by people trying to make decisions before they have sufficient knowledge on which to base a decision. Why worry about the future. Just imagine as to what if we just acted like everything was easy and there was nothing very serious about it to come in future. Worry often gives a small thing a big shadow and its surrounding do frightened with more scary things. Why worry about tomorrow; concentrate on today happening as for tomorrow will worry about itself. Each day has its own worries and troubles.

If there is not any solution to the some problem then do not waste time worrying about it. And if there is a solution to the problem then why waste time worrying about it. Worry will never rob tomorrow of its sorrows, but will only deny today of its meaning happiness and joys. Worrying is actually a form of superstition and creates false images in our mind and that is the main reason and cause which makes and leads us to this point of imagination. A human being can survive almost anything, as long as he or she sees the end in sight. If something bad or good is to happen it is sure to happen, whether we worry or not. Let us put our energy into today and stop worrying about the future and past. We should not foresee trouble, or worry about what may never happen as past is dead and gone forever and future is uncertain and yet to come. The basic facts we should know about worry.

The basic techniques to analyze worry and how to break the worry habit before it breaks us. These are the simple ways where we can concentrate and get rid of worries prevailing in our thoughts. Annalise worry to see and get the reasons and facts of worry. To avoid reoccurrence of worries, concentrate on prayers as prayers are the best source of remedies of the prevailing worries. The more you pray, the less you'll panic. The more you worship, the less you worry. There is nothing that wastes the body like worry, and anyone who has any faith in God should need not to worry about anything whatsoever is to happen in future. We ought to know the basic fundamental of analyzing worries.

Worries create unnecessary thoughts and these are caused by people going in for unwanted decisions, fore hand not even knowing as to when a good decision is made and not even having sufficient knowledge about it. We must first study and after carefully weighing all the facts than only come to a powerful decision. Simply making castles in the air won't solve our problems but add more to our vows. Anxiety and worry can go hand in hand. When anxiety grabs the mind, it is self-perpetuating. Your mind gets clogged with numerous with buts and ifs. Do not worry about your life. Worries are repetitive thoughts associated with feelings of anxiety in anticipation of some negative future event. Yet anxious feelings and the worries that lead to them can prove helpful. It becomes a difficult problem if you are constantly anxious as it will become a hindrance to your everyday life, rather than motivate you to some good and better things. Never worry alone. Worrisome thoughts reproduce faster so one of the most powerful ways to stop the spiral of worry is simply to disclose the worry to a friend. What you will eat or drink; or about your body, what you will wear. If you know that the circumstance is beyond your control or power change than revise it to your liking. Just try to put a stop-less order on your worries. Don't permit little things which become insects of life to ruin your happiness. Co-operate with the inevitable. Decide just how much anxiety a thing may be worth and refuse to give in anymore. All the happiness is not given in one go it comes slowly and slowly. If your worries center on, an important relationship in your life, pay special attention to remain positive and be happy. To keep yourself happy, treat your worried thoughts as valuable signals.

How to keep from worrying about criticism? Simply unjust criticism is often a disguised compliment. It often means that you have aroused jealousy and envy. Let's keep a record of the fool things we have done and criticize ourselves. The utmost cause of worry is your state of depression. Worries are there to motivate information-gathering and problem-solving. Depression is the inability to construct a future. Depression is inertia. That's the thing about depression: But depression is so insidious, and it compounds daily, that it's impossible to ever see the end. Depressed people think they know themselves, but maybe they only know depression. There are no hopeless than this to get depressed. Our attitude towards suffering and depression becomes very important because it can affect how we cope with suffering when it arises. Depression is nourished by a lifetime of un grieved and unforgiving causes. Never worry about your heart till it stops beating. How can you deal with anxiety? You might try what when you did. A person worried so much that he decided to hire someone to do his worrying for him. Times will change for the better when you change. Worry is a misuse of the imagination. Worry is most often a prideful way of thinking that you have more control over life and its circumstances than you actually do. To keep yourself happy, treat your worried thoughts as valuable signals. These are the fundamental facts you should be familiar about worries. A huge factor to stay happy is to cater your worries around, an important relationship in your life and pay special attention sustaining positive relationships. Worries are there to motivate information gathering and problem-solving.

Make your mind firm and do come to a positive decision as come what we will not allow the worries to entire our mind and soul. Once a decision is carefully reached we should get busy carrying out our decisions and should not bother about all the anxieties that are about to come. When we, or any of our colleagues or associates, are about to worry about a problem, we must write it out and think of the following questions: Instead of worrying about what people say of you, why not spend time trying to accomplish something they will admire.

What if we just acted like everything was easy? How would your life be different if you stopped worrying about things we can't control and started focusing on the things we can? Let today be the day. You free yourself from fruitless worry, seize the day and take effective action on things you can change.

LEAVE WORRIES NOW
BE HAPPY ENJOY LIFE
CHAPTER 18

HAVE POSITIVITY WITHIN US

You may feel largely uncomfortable, when worries attack your thoughts and mind which makes worrying about a situation an easier option to get depressed and diffused. While you are consuming more worries you are far too busy to do anything else to fix the real problem and would rather find it hard to get into a smart solution. Thus resulting in a fact that you spend your evenings worrying only without even bothering to find some time to search a new job. You get nothing out of worrying except only to think and cry. Another cause of getting worried is the attachment with which your inner soul gets attracted to. Attachment brings worry. If you have a problem and you come up with the answer, you stop worrying immediately. Our minds can be dishonest, persuading us that we are worrying about something, when our deepest fear is entirely different. No-one likes to admit that they've chosen to worry. The first step is to write down your worries, which will help you make sense of them, and then decide on one small step you can take towards a solution. But to be very true no man in this world is free of obstacles or difficulties. Don't make worry your habit. Break this habit and stop all the negative and panic thoughts provoking your mind all the time. If you can't change the past, but you must not ruin the present by worrying about the future. Joy is what happens to us when we allow ourselves to recognize how good things really are.

When we feel worried and depressed, we need to consciously form a smile on our faces and act upbeat until the happy feeling becomes genuine reality. Feelings of depression and hopelessness and or anger are even tougher to cope with on a consistent basis. When you are worried, you not only hurt yourself, but the limited support systems that are still holding on your mind but making you to get more and more worried and nothing is achieved in terms of success except the re-carnation of worries and worries. Your actions breed confidence and courage. If you want to conquer fear, anger and worry do not sit ideal and just think about it. Let our deep worrying become advance thinking and planning. If you look into your own mind and heart, and you find nothing wrong there, what is there to worry about? Practically nothing what is there to fear about and again nothing? So why worry unnecessarily and make your present and future dark.

Negative Thoughts Provoke Our Minds

Negative thought which are provoking our mind, about the uncertainties and the negativities, as to what will happen tomorrow creates unnecessary worries and worries are repetitive thoughts associated with feelings of anxiety in anticipation of some negative future event which may end in a failure. Whether the worries are about financial crisis, family problems, work, health or any topic of concern, the anxious feelings and negative thoughts produced are always distinctly unpleasant. Annalise positive thinking and stop worry over petty matters. Worrying will carry tomorrow's load with today's strength.

Worry will not empty tomorrow of its sorrows, but it tends to empty today of its power and strength. Worries make you to move into tomorrow ahead of time. Half the worry in the world is caused by people trying to make decisions before they have sufficient knowledge on which to base a decision. Their negative thoughts pressurize them to be away from the positivity in their lives as they fail and do not analysis on positive. Why worry about the future. Just imagine as to what if we just acted like everything was easy and there was nothing very serious about it to come in future. Worry often gives a small thing a big shadow and its surrounding do frightened with more scary things. Why worry about tomorrow; concentrate on today happening as for tomorrow will worry about itself. Each day has its own worries and troubles. Always think positive. If there is not any solution to the some problem then do not waste time worrying about it. And if there is a solution to the problem then why waste time worrying about it. Act fast be positive generate positive thinking worries will automatically vanish in the air. But if you tend to worry they will never rob tomorrow of its sorrows, but will only deny today of its meaning happiness and joys. Negative thoughts only produce worries and worrying is actually a form of superstition and creates false images in our mind and that is the main reason and cause which makes and leads us to this point of imagination. A human being can survive almost anything, as long as he or she sees the end in sight and starts analyzing his positive thoughts. We must not forgot that something bad or good is to happen it is sure to happen, whether we worry or not. Let us put our energy into today and stop worrying about the future and past.

We should not foresee trouble, or worry about what may never happen as past is dead and gone forever and future is uncertain and yet to come. Positive Thinking will ward off everything and bring happiness in our lives. The basic facts we should know about worry. The basic techniques to analyze worry and how to break the worry habit before it breaks us. These are the simple ways where we can concentrate and get rid of worries prevailing in our thoughts.

Think Positive and Pray- Why Worry?

Annalise positive thinking by annualizing worry you get to see and get the reasons and facts of worry. To avoid reoccurrence of worries, concentrate on prayers as prayers are the best source of remedies of the prevailing worries. Think Positive and Pray. The more you pray, the less you'll panic. The more you worship, the less you worry.

Generate Positive Thinking

There is nothing that wastes the body like worry, and anyone who has any faith in God should need not to worry about anything whatsoever is to happen in future. Positive thinking is the creation of good imagination. We must first study and after carefully weighing all the facts than only come to a powerful decision. Simply making castles in the air won't solve our problems but add more to our vows. Anxiety and worry can go hand in hand. When anxiety grabs the mind, it is self-perpetuating. Your mind gets clogged with numerous with buts and ifs. Do not worry about your life.

Worries are repetitive thoughts associated with feelings of anxiety in anticipation of some negative future event. Yet anxious feelings and the worries that lead to them can prove helpful. It becomes a difficult problem if you are constantly anxious to know as to the happening of the future. It will become a hindrance to your everyday life, rather than motivate you to some good and better things. Worrisome thoughts reproduce faster so one of the most powerful ways to stop the spiral of worry is simply to disclose the worry to a friend. What you eat or drink; or about your body, what you will wear will add to negativity may discard positive thinking.

Happiness comes with Positive Thinking.

If you know that the circumstance is beyond your control or power change than revise it to your liking. Just try to put a stop-less order on your worries. Don't permit little things which become insects of life to ruin your happiness. Co-operate with the inevitable. Decide just how much anxiety a thing may be worth and refuse to give in anymore. All the happiness is not given in one go it comes slowly and slowly with positive thinking.

Have worry under your control. If your worries center around, pay special attention to remain positive and be happy. Keep yourself happy, treat your worried thoughts as valuable signals. How to keep from worrying about criticism? Simply unjust criticism and think positively and do often discard a bad compliment. It often means that you have aroused jealousy and envy. Let's keep a record of the fool things we have done and stop criticizing ourselves.

Cause of Worry is Negative Thinking- Think Positive

The utmost cause of worry is our negative thinking as it leads us to the state of depression. Worries are there to motivate us and not a mere source of information-gathering and problems. Dejection and Depression is the inability to construct a future. Depression is inertia. That's the thing about depression: But depression is so insidious, and it compounds daily, that it's impossible to ever see the end. Depressed people think they know themselves, but maybe they only know depression. There are no hopeless than this to get depressed. They never even attempt to think positive.

Times will change for the better-Think Positive

Our negative thinking and attitude towards suffering and depression becomes very important because it can affect how we cope with suffering when it arises. Depression is nourished by a lifetime of un-grieved and unforgiven causes. Never worry about your heart till it stops beating. How can you deal with anxiety? You might try what when you did. A person worried so much that he decided to hire someone to do his worrying for him. Times will change for the better when you change. Worry is a misuse of the imagination. Worry is most often a prideful way of thinking that you have more control over life and its circumstances than you actually do. Positive Thinking leads your way to good and happiness. An art of Good and Happy Living. Neglect worries keep yourself happy, treat your worried thoughts as valuable signals. These are the fundamental facts you should be familiar about worries.

A huge factor to stay happy is to cater your worries around, an important relationship in your life and pay special attention sustaining positive relationships. Worries are there to motivate information gathering and problem-solving. Make your mind firm and do come to a positive decision as come what we will not allow the worries to entire our mind and soul. Once a decision is carefully reached we should get busy carrying out our decisions and should not bother about all the anxieties that are about to come. When we, or any of our colleagues or associates, are about to worry about a problem, we must write it out and think positively of the questions: Instead of worrying about what people say of you, why not spend time trying to accomplish something they will admire. What if we just acted like everything was easy? How would your life be different if you stopped worrying about things we can't control and started focusing on the things we can? Let today be the day. You free yourself from fruitless worry, seize the day and take effective action on things you can change. We would change ourselves for the betterment if we start thinking in positive terms. Positive thinking is what is required of us and simply worrying about the future things or as to what will happen in the next moment will certainly deprive us of good and happy living that we are about gather or get in the next hour.

LEAVE WORRIES NOW
BE HAPPY ENJOY LIFE

CHAPTER 19

STAY OPEN TO LAUGHTER AND HUMOUR

Even when you are facing challenges, it is important to stay open to laughter and humor. Sometimes, simply recognizing the potential humor in a situation can lessen your stress and brighten your outlook. Seeking out sources of humor such as watching a funny sitcom or reading jokes online can help you think more positive thoughts. We need to know and realize that nobody is perfect or flawless. If we try to change the way we look, talk and behave just to please others, and show our pride we will gradually become such a person that we ourselves won't recognize each other and would start and create unnecessary worries within us and our surrounding without being positive and will not start to live happily. We ought to stop worrying over unnecessary things be positive and live without fear happily. As a result, negative thoughts can creep into your mind. While you know that thinking positively is better for your state of mind, you might be surprised to learn that it can also be good for your health. We need to understand that what people think of us is their concern, and not ours. If they think about us to be, too reticent or proud, it's really not our business. If every time we happen to meet some new fellows, we may wonder and imagine as what they think of us, and with this feeling in us we will never be able to live a trouble-free and hassle free life. We are bound to fall into the trap of unnecessary worries denying us the startup of new and the happy living life.

We must think rationally. Is it in our hands or can we control what others think about us? Simply we need to ignore them If we cannot, and live our lives the way we want to and find the ways to leave worries aside and start living a happy life. Let us make our way to happy living.

Positive Thinking with Positive Attitudes.

Positive thinking is not about putting on a pair of rose-colored glasses and ignoring all the negative things you will encounter in life. That approach can be just as devastating as ignoring the positive and only focusing on the negative. Balance, with a healthy dose of realism, is the key. It is a well-known fact that attitude decides how a natives or persons copes up with the day to day events of life. Attitude is what a influence a person's reaction to a situation in life is. It sets the emotional undertone for a person to his likes or dislikes a situation even before he is acquainted with it. Positive attitude is a quality that is second to none in a human being. Though we attach so much importance to this attitude, as we grow into teenage and adult years we find ourselves becoming ungrateful or taking things for granted. We lose touch with the very same qualities that we instill in our children. We take for granted our life, our health, our families, the people in our lives, the things that our loved ones do for us to make our lives easier and things that we possess. The attitude of positive speaks a lot about a person. It denotes about changing negative attitudes and making positive thinking a positive attitude a good habit. Thinking positively and a positive attitude help us to appreciate and value ourselves, our potential and all that we have. It ensures that we do not take our abilities for granted. It makes us look at ourselves as special people with a special set of abilities and potential. It banishes the feelings of inadequacy and insecurity that arises from unfair comparisons with others.

It helps us to appreciate people for who they are and not magnify what they are not and their little flaws. It drives away prejudice and makes us approach life with an open mind. It predisposes us to react to the daily events of life in a positive manner and help us to look at the brighter side of life. Make us optimistic. It gives hope and helps us look forward to life with anticipation. We need to know that positive thinking takes the focus away from what we don't have, to appreciating and making good use of what we have. It is closely connected to our emotional wellbeing and happiness. We feel loved and at peace with ourselves for a major part of our lives when we make this attitude ours. This adds and helps us to get rid of greed, amenity, bitterness, jealousy, and promotes a healthy and nurturing attitude towards others, which in turn gets reciprocated and we feel the sense of healthy living. We attach so much importance to this attitude of gratitude that when our children fail to thank someone, we insist that they do it. That is what is needed to be avoided from time to time. We expect this in return from others when we help them or give them a gift. We call a person discourteous and rude when they do not say thank us in return. On the face of it we ought to know that a positive is not an attitude of being satisfied and content, that you never want to do anything, anymore. This is an attitude that makes you feel good about who you are, what you do, and what your potentials are. This attitude impels you to utilize all that you are endowed with as a person, to achieve the highest possible goals. When we have this attitude, we are able to work without any external pressure to perform but there is sufficient pressure and motivation from within. The possessing of positive thinking is like any other habit, so we need to follow the routine of habit formation here as well. You will win new friends and admirers without having to impress them or conform to the pressure of doing things their way.

You will be bubbling with life and the joie de vivre. You will be rearing to go and accomplish all you can with your new found confidence. The best part of adopting the 'positive thinking and a positive attitude of gratitude is that, you will be able to enjoy the smallest pleasures of nature with a heightened sense of satisfaction and awe. I can see and watch a beautiful flower and carry that joy in my mind for future enjoyment with a clear positive habit. I can go back to work freshen and can use it as an object to meditate on when I feel stressed. Let us be clear that a positive is not an attitude of being satisfied and content, that you never want to do anything, anymore. This is an attitude that makes you feel good about who you are, what you do, and what your potentials are. This attitude impels you to utilize all that you are endowed with as a person, to achieve the highest possible goals. When we have this attitude, we are able to work without any external pressure to perform but there is sufficient pressure and motivation from within. The habit of positive thinking is like any other habit, so we need to follow the routine of habit formation here as well.

LEAVE WORRIES NOW
BE HAPPY ENJOY LIFE

CHAPTER 20

WHY DISAPPOINTMENT

Being a positive thinker is not about ignoring reality in favor of aspirational thoughts. It is more about taking a proactive approach to your life. Instead of feeling hopeless or overwhelmed, positive thinking allows you to tackle life's challenges by looking for effective ways to resolve conflict and come up with creative solutions to problems. It might not be easy, but the positive impact it will have on your mental, emotional, and physical health will be well-worth it. At time we may think that there is no road is left for us from where we can achieve the happiness of our lives. We may also feel that life has become terrible for us to live and we are carrying new hope that someone would come to rescue us. There may be chances that someone who was there with us before might have held on to us when we were on the dark side of the life. What if when everything goes wrong and all the doors of happiness are closed our live becomes a silent. It is a quite common and we are aware of a marvelous proverb that Life itself is a stage and we all are the performers, performing different acts assigned to us by our almighty power. We should not forget as to what is in our possession?, if it is to fulfill our duties towards our responsibility and do whatever is correct and is allowed by us in our life?. We should not forget that happiness in life comes through the doors of positive thoughts; we need to have them first. If one door happen to close, another opens, in the event only when we are confident and optimistic. We have so many reasons to cry and at the same time plenty of reasons to smile as well.

Similarly, happiness does not stand for anything, but is on our way of thinking that how do we keep ourselves happy in life. Failure and disappointment are part of our life. The only thing is that we need to face and solve the problem is by keeping our dreams and hope alive be it a reason that success and happiness will come our way again. There are quite a number of reasons to believe that for a successful and happy life the mystery surrounding it lies in our interests, and good memory which is the basis of our interest, power of desire and aim, keeping ourselves smiling and the doubt free character which is the foremost important reason for a successful and happy life. If we possess one solid unselfish and doubt free character within ourselves we would be quite happy and successful. The experience has taught us that we should buy some strength, hope and positivity from our loved ones to help ourselves in such a situation rather than surrendering as life is a precious gift of God and is equipped with full of joy and happiness if we help ourselves in these critical moments we can live with considerable optimism. Now let's us imagine that we are not feeling at our best today, and we are having thoughts that could be classified as negative. We shouldn't be thinking such negative thoughts. We don't like the negative thoughts. We ought to know that negative thoughts are stressful, demoralizing and depressing. We shouldn't aim to have negative thoughts at all. Often we feel uncomfortable because we think we have to say or do something in response to another person's words. When we find ourselves thinking this way, it helps enormously to take a few moments to check inside and notice what we are feeling. We are deeply depressed that negativity has governed us and has taken a deep root in our minds. So, let's imagine that you have chosen to focus on your negative thinking with regards to school.

The next step is to spend a little bit of time each day evaluating your own thoughts. When you find yourself thinking critical thoughts about yourself, take a moment to pause and reflect. While you might be upset about getting a bad grade on an exam, is berating yourself really the best approach? Is there any way to put a positive spin on the situation? While you might not have done well on this exam, at least you have a better indication of how to structure your study time for the next big test. However, despite of all these good thoughts which are embodied to us by the almighty fail to revive these unwanted circumstances that lead us to sorrow and difficulties and a situation where we do not know what is correct and good for us and what is wrong for us. We should always remember that, "Life is there, where there is hope". That single thing that remains in our hands is to find out ways to know how to overcome these worries of our life at that very moment when all doors are closed for us which means that whatever situation is there, we must not give up hope. We must fight because there have been always a chance that with good faith and hard work we can turn the odds in our favor. It is often said that it is very easy to advice but when it comes to us, things go out of our control and we fail to suggest a way out for ourselves. We fall into the trap of unnecessary worries and elope ourselves with negative thoughts. We feel better when somebody else is facing some difficulty but when it comes to us we fail to gather that faith, will power and the words of strength. Being a positive thinker is not about ignoring reality in favor of aspirational thoughts. It is more about taking a proactive approach to your life. Instead of feeling hopeless or overwhelmed, positive thinking allows you to tackle life's challenges by looking for effective ways to resolve conflict and come up with creative solutions to problems. It might not be easy, but the positive impact it will have on your mental, emotional, and physical health will be well-worth it. It takes practice; lots of practice.

This is not a step-by-step process that you can complete and be done with. Instead, it involves a lifelong commitment to looking inside yourself and being willing to challenge negative thoughts and make positive changes. It is a common fact that no one in this world is free of obstacles or difficulties. If all the openings of happiness are shut for us and we have to overcome that and have no way to come out, but to survive lest we must have to learn to swim out of the sorrows because this is what is called life and sorrow free living. There are lot more examples and in many other situations, where we will find that how we could have faced and fought with our sorrows and difficulties of life when there was no hope left in our lives. When the power of will is at the worst and each one of us knows that the one who is gone never comes back. Neither a thousands of words would not be enough to bring him back nor a million tears, because each and every moment, eyes would only shed tears , mind would remain tensed and we would be simply surrounded by worries and the life seems to have been vanished. Life is ever expanding, contraction is death. As commonly said by big saints that the self- seeking man who is looking after his personal comforts and leading a lazy life for himself there would be no room for him even in the hell and he simply have lost the power of his will. One cannot do anything without it. We fail only when we do not try very hard to achieve the power and faith within us. As soon as we lose faith, death comes in our way and we are surrounds by all the evils and stupid worries of the world. The secret and history of every successful man is to have, good confidence, faith and strength behind him and that remain the right cause of his single success in life. Unselfishness plays a very vital role in his life. He may not have been perfectly unselfish, yet he was tending towards it. If he had been perfectly unselfish, he would have been as great a success.

The degree of unselfishness marks the degree of success everywhere and he leads to be successful man without fear worries and selfishness. Therefore creation of positivity in life is utmost necessary to enjoy the special gift of God to us. The love for God and worshipping God adds to one common thing the immense faith in Him. There may be different beliefs and ways to worship God in different communities, places and religions, but one thing remains the same and that is the Love of God for all of us. Our world is full of odds and evens, happiness and sorrows, fulfilment and emptiness. And these are all created by the Almighty. However, the most beautiful Gift of God, is Human, which is such a mystery driven by Him which could hardly be defined or explained in depth. We know that life cannot be foreseen. Life is not a bed of roses. Life is a battle field and not a bed of roses as every man on earth has to struggle very hard in making his life happy. If aim of our life is to stay happy and let others to be happy, we will be happy and remembered by all. But no one will actually remember us for the wealth we have gained, or success we have achieved. I have no aim in life. Summary living with no purpose in life is just like a feather moving towards the wind. Life is such a special gift of Almighty and it is not gifted by Him to use it the way we like or love to. The actual path shown by Him needs to be followed by us for us to reach the peak of betterment every moment. We need to have some positive attitude to look at it comfortably but at the same time having a positive mental attitude does not mean banishing all negative thoughts and people from your life. One and another one arises.

LEAVE WORRIES NOW
BE HAPPY ENJOY LIFE

CHAPTER 21

NOT HAPPY - WHY?

If you are interested in getting more success and happiness

If you are interested in getting more success and happiness within you, focus on all the ways as if you have already attained success. You need to focus on the thing and create a happy live within you. If you want love and affection, focus on all the people and the abundance of love that you have to give to them. If we want to have greater health, focus on all the ways that we are healthy, thus creating and delivering a good life within you. You need to admit that there are problems that you cannot change. But you can change the way of your thinking if you identify the main reason of the problem. And if you acknowledge the facts, that you have been negative or inactive in finding a solution to the problem, probably this will make it easier for you to become positive thus creating a new lease of life within you. It will make your life easier to lead a good and sweet life.

You must try to make goals

You must try to make goals. Making goals can give you a more positive outlook on life. People often tend to get bored with life and get the feeling that they are stuck to negative things which the result they often get the feeling of being depressed. Setting a direction for yourself and a goal would surely help you to move forward.

Mental attitude that can bring you peace and happiness

If you expecting to succeed, and are not afraid of failure, you have the best chance of staying positive and can create a very positive life within you. When you, or any of your associates, are tempted to worry about a problem, write out the solution and a definite answer to it. This helps a positive feeling to generate within you making you very positive to have a good living.

Another thing you need to understand is that there are several ways to cultivate a mental attitude that can bring you peace and happiness and can carnage a good life within you. More of it if you fill your mind with thoughts of peace, courage, health, and hope, your life will be easy to live. You would get a happy feeling of life and mind if you let yourself to forget your own unhappiness, by trying to create a little happiness for others. You are best to yourself and to others.

The first step is to write down your worries

The first step is to write down your worries, which will help you make sense of them, and then decide on one small step you can take towards a solution. But to be very true no man in this world is free of obstacles or difficulties. Don't make worry your habit. Break this habit and stop all the negative and panic thoughts provoking your mind all the time. If you can't change the past, but you must not ruin the present by worrying about the future. Joy is what happens to us when we allow ourselves to recognize how good things really are. When we feel worried and depressed, we need to consciously form a smile on our faces and act upbeat until the happy feeling becomes genuine reality. Happiness is what is needed most. What makes to lead a happy life is not to get trapped into unnecessary unwanted worries and negative thoughts.

Don't create the feeling of depression and anger.

Feelings of depression and hopelessness and or anger are even tougher to cope with on a consistent basis. When you are worried, you not only hurt yourself, but the limited support systems that are still holding on your mind but making you to get more and more worried and nothing is achieved in terms of success except the re-carnation of worries and worries thus leading you to be unhappy and worried all the time. Your actions breed confidence and courage. If you want to conquer fear, anger and worry do not sit ideal and just think about it. Let our deep worrying become advance thinking and planning.

If you look into your own mind and heart, and you find nothing wrong there, what is there to worry about? Practically nothing what is there to fear about and again nothing? So why worry unnecessarily and make your present and future dark. Neglect all those which make your life unhappy.

Why being a negative person?

Why being a negative person and what do you get out of it being a depression dejected and sad man.? Why not turn your thoughts to be a positive person simply it is a question of tilting your mind towards a positive side of thing. See both the aspects of a situation and ways the pros and cons of both the sides and try to abolish the negativity in you. Be positive strong and you will remain happy for ever. We all have different roles that we play in the lives of people we love and care about. Our actions and how well we play our part has a direct influence on their life, so we better get in there and give our best performance. Tell them with how much you care in the capacity that you're in. At the end of the day, money is just a means to an end. Nothing more. If you're grinding and struggling to make ends meet and buried under piles of debt, that's pretty stressful.

Once you have your basic needs met though, more money only makes you happier up to a certain point. Money cannot buy you happiness. You need to generate it yourself. Someone will always be better than you at something, but it does not matter. Be inspired by them, using it to push yourself further, and nothing more. If they can do it, why cannot you?

Are you are interested in getting more happiness?.

If you are interested in getting more happiness focus on all the ways as if you have already attained success. You need to focus on the thing and create a live within you. If you want love and affection, focus on all the people and the abundance of love that you have to give to them.

Worrisome thoughts reproduce faster.

Worrisome thoughts reproduce faster so one of the most powerful ways to stop the spiral of worry is simply to disclose the worry to a friend. Practice happy gratitude daily. Take three minutes at the end of your day to chill and write down a small list of the things that can make you smile, laugh, or that you're glad are a part of your life. There's something to be grateful about, especially when you look down at that list and realize that a lot of people have it worse off than you do and could use a few of those things. Simply being an optimist will not solve all your problems, but what's the alternative is to keep your mind and heart cool and always have happy and positive feeling and think that life is to live happily. There isn't much sense in being anything else. If you're constantly filling your head with negative thoughts, odds are they'll lead you straight towards negative actions, self-doubt and increase the general happiness of life isn't a cool place to live at all. Think of each setback as a challenge to see the positive, spin the situation back around, making it better than it was before and start living in a good and sweet manner.

What do we get out of unhappiness?

We may feel largely uncomfortable, when worries attack our thoughts and mind. While we are consuming more worries we are far too busy to do anything else to fix the real problem and would rather find it hard to get into a smart solution. Thus resulting in a fact that you spend your evenings worrying only without even bothering to find some time to know its cause We get nothing out of worrying except only to think and cry and become unhappy. We do not get anything out of unhappiness. Another thing is that we may feel largely uncomfortable, when worries attack our thoughts and mind which makes worrying about a situation an easier option to get depressed and diffused. While we are consuming more worries we are far too busy to do anything else to fix the real problem and would rather find it hard to get into a smart solution.

Thus resulting in a fact that we spend our evenings worrying only without even bothering to find some time to search a sweet happiness within us. Negative thought which are provoking our mind, about the uncertainties and the negativities, as to what will happen tomorrow creates unnecessary worries and worries are repetitive thoughts associated with feelings of anxiety in anticipation of some negative future event which may end in a failure.

Negative thoughts create unnecessary worries

Whether the worries are about financial crisis, family problems, work, health or any topic of concern, the anxious feelings and negative thoughts produced are always distinctly unpleasant thus making us unhappy all the time. We get nothing being a negative and unhappy man. We must not forget that if we tend to worry they will never rob tomorrow of its sorrows, but will only deny today of its meaning happiness and joys.

Negative thoughts only produce worries and worrying is actually a form of superstition and creates false images in our mind and that is the main reason and cause which makes and leads us to this point of imagination. A human being can survive almost anything, as long as he or she sees the end in sight, starts analyzing his positive thoughts and starts analyzing his unhappiness.

LEAVE WORRIES NOW
BE HAPPY ENJOY LIFE

CHAPTER 22

DISCARD NEGATIVE THINKING

You may also feel that life has become terrible for you to live and you are carrying no hope that someone would be there to rescue you. Happiness is your own choice and decision. Each of us can be as happy as we make up our minds to be. We can, if we want, fill up our days with positive attitude chatter and laughter. To be happy, we need to concentrate only on happy thoughts. The ghosts of the past have to be exorcised. You may be working in any field, the key to success is your outlook. Sometimes you may think that no road is left for you from where you can achieve the happiness of life. There may be chances that someone who was there with you before might hold on to you when you are on the dark side of the life. The experience has taught us that we should buy some strength, hope and positive ness from our loved ones to help ourselves in such a situation rather than surrendering as life is a precious gift of God and is equipped with full of joy and happiness if we help ourselves in these critical moments and live with considerable optimism. Happiness in life comes through the doors of positive thoughts; we do not even realize which one is left open. We have so many reasons to cry and at the same time plenty of reasons to smile as well. Keeping our dreams and hope alive might be a reason that success and happiness will come our way again. We ought to know that happiness alone does not stand for anything, but it is on our way of thinking that how do we keep ourselves happy in life.

Ending up our lives does not lead us to our destination but of course proves we are supposed to be cowards who know not to unfold the doors of belief in God and in ourselves. Failure and disappointment are part of our life. The only thing is that we need to face and solve the problem. We must not forget to believe in God whatever our situation may be, we would be taken away from Him by the difficulties, in order that we bow down and surrender. But if our faith is strong enough we will not be let down, rather we would break the knees of sorrows and force it to die and lead happy lives. We should not surrender but must find out ways to come out of our worries, anxieties and difficulties. We ought not to indulge ourselves into the darkness of the room but find out the doors to free ourselves from unnecessary fear and worries. We must belief in ourselves and our hearts, and believe in the ones who love us and not the ones whom we love. We must not fall on the negative side of a thing. It is the real time when you keep on revealing the truth of our lives and relations, do not fall on the reverse side but think how good it was that because of the hard times of our lives we could well judge about them. We should always try to be positive and should think that whatever is happening, it is the positive side or consequence of that incident in would be on the positive side of our imagination. With all these thoughts, I would request my readers to implement some good thoughts in their life that would make things easier to be tackled by them. We should accept the situation and fight it with more determination. In this world nothing is good or bad and only thinking makes it so. We ought to know that advice from people around us will help us to overcome from the any drastic situation. Also we have to always minimize the stress as it gives nothing but takes away joy and happiness from our lives. And finally we need to take things casually and fight with it seriously.

The next morning after all, will surely come with fresh air to breathe the new hopes in us with the brightness of the sun. A clear minded person looks for good qualities in the other person, whereas a negative mind always looks for the fault in the other person, whereas a negative mind always looks for the fault. An optimist goes forward keeping in mind the past, a pessimist thinks of the future and reverts back to the past. In fact negative thoughts are our greatest enemies. Experience the happiness in all circumstances by maintaining better relationships. How about understanding that sadness cannot touch a person with a positive attitude? The capability increases as It boosts up patience and confidence. It increases the decision of making power. Creative way of thoughts appears in the mind. Positive thoughts teach the art of finding solutions to any problem. Optimism is something what we do. Anxiety and other negative emotions are known to be detrimental to the body, especially to our immune systems, and having an optimistic nature seems to protect against those effects. People who are supposed to be optimistic, about their future, behaving differently. They do exercise, do not indulge in in smoking and often follow a good and better diet. Whenever we are unhappy, if we analyze the reason for our unhappiness, it is because life is not matching our expectations.

LEAVE WORRIES NOW
BE HAPPY ENJOY LIFE

CHAPTER 23

STOP WORRYING AND START LIVING

At time we may think that there is no road is left for us from where we can achieve the happiness of our lives. We may also feel that life has become terrible for us to live and we are carrying new hope that someone would come to rescue us. There may be chances that someone who was there with us before might have held on to us when we were on the dark side of the life.

It is important for us to stay open to laughter and humor.

Even when we are facing challenges, it is important for us to stay open to laughter and humor. Sometimes, simply recognizing the potential humor in a situation can lessen our stress and brighten our outlook. Seeking out sources of humor such as watching a funny sitcom or reading jokes online can help us to think more positively. The experience has taught us that we should buy some strength, hope and positive ness from our loved ones to help ourselves in such a situation rather than surrendering as life is a precious gift of God and is equipped with full of joy and happiness if we help ourselves in these critical moments and live with considerable optimism. Happiness in life comes through the doors of positive thoughts; we do not even realize which one is left open.

We have so many reasons to cry and at the same time plenty of reasons to smile as well.

Keeping our dreams and hope alive might be a reason that success and happiness will come our way again. We ought to know that happiness alone does not stand for anything, but it is on our way of thinking that how do we keep ourselves happy in life. Ending up our lives does not lead us to our destination but of course proves we are supposed to be cowards who know not to unfold the doors of belief in God and in ourselves. But if our faith is strong enough we will not be let down, rather we would break the knees of sorrows and force it to die and lead happy lives.

We must find out ways to come out of our worries, anxieties and difficulties.

We should not surrender but must find out ways to come out of our worries, anxieties and difficulties. We ought not to indulge ourselves into the darkness of the room but find out the doors to free ourselves from unnecessary fear and worries. We must belief in ourselves and our hearts, and believe in the ones who love us and not the ones whom we love. We must not fall on the negative side of a thing. It is the real time when we keep on revealing the truth of our lives and relations. We should always try to be happy and should think that whatever is happening, it is the positive side. We should accept the situation and fight it with more determination. We must find out ways to come out of our worries, anxieties and difficulties in order for us to lead a happy sweet and good life.

Negative thoughts are our greatest enemies.

We ought to know that advice from people around us will help us to overcome from the any drastic situation. Also we have to always minimize the stress as it gives nothing but takes away joy and happiness from our lives. And finally we need to take things casually and fight with it seriously. A clear minded person looks for good qualities in the other person, whereas a negative mind always looks for the fault in the other person, whereas a negative mind always looks for the fault. An optimist goes forward keeping in mind the past, a pessimist thinks of the future and reverts back to the past. In fact negative thoughts are our greatest enemies. Experience the happiness in all circumstances by maintaining better relationships.

We need to analyise the reason for our unhappiness.

Whenever we are unhappy, if we analyze the reason for our unhappiness, it is because life is not matching our desires and expectations. We need to know and realize that nobody is perfect or flawless. If we try to change the way we look, talk and behave just to please others, and show our pride we will gradually become such a person that we ourselves won't recognize each other and would start and create unnecessary worries within us and our surrounding without being positive and will not start to live happily. We ought to stop worrying over unnecessary things be positive and live without fear. Living happily is the master key to all problems and worries. Forgot worries discard all problems take them lightly and behave as nothing serious has happened. This way we are sure to overcome all problems and lead a happy life. We need to understand that what people think of us is their concern, and not ours.

If they think about us to be, too reticent or proud, it's really not our business. If every time we happen to meet some new fellows, we may wonder and imagine as what they think of us, and with this feeling in us we will never be able to live a trouble-free and hassle free life. We are bound to fall into the trap of unnecessary worries denying us the startup of new and the happy living life.

Positive attitude is a quality of happy living.

We must think rationally. Is it in our hands or can we control what others think about us? Simply we need to ignore them, if we cannot, and live our lives the way we want to and find the ways to leave worries aside and start living a happy life. Let us make our way to happy living. It is a well-known fact that attitude decides how a natives or persons copes up with the day to day events of life. Attitude is the main influence a person's reaction to a situation in life. It sets the emotional undertone for a person to his likes or dislikes a situation even before he is acquainted with it. Positive attitude is a quality of happy living which is second to none in a human being. We acknowledge our children to say a big thank you from the time to time irrespective they being very little, we teach them to be grateful for everything that they receive. We attach so much importance to this attitude of gratitude that when our children fail to thank someone, we insist that they do it. That is what is needed to be avoided from time to time. We expect this in return from others when we help them or give them a gift. We call a person discourteous and rude when they do not say thank us in return.

Though we attach so much importance to this attitude, as we grow into teenage and adult years we find ourselves becoming ungrateful or taking things for granted. We lose touch with the very same qualities that we instill in our children. We take for granted our life, our health, our families, the people in our lives, the things that our loved ones do for us to make our lives easier and things that we possess.

The attitude of positive or happy living speaks a lot about a person.

It denotes about changing negative attitudes and making positive thinking a positive a good habit. Thinking positively and a positive attitude help us to appreciate and value ourselves, our potential and all that we have. It ensures that we do not take our abilities for granted. It makes us look at ourselves as special people with a special set of abilities and potential. It banishes the feelings of inadequacy and insecurity that arises from unfair comparisons with others. It helps us to appreciate people for who they are and not magnify what they are not and their little flaws. It drives away prejudice and makes us approach life with an open mind. It predisposes us to react to the daily events of life in a positive manner and help us to look at the brighter side of life. Make us optimistic. It gives hope and helps us look forward to life with anticipation making our lives happier and happier day by day. We need to know that positive thinking takes the focus away from what we don't have, to appreciating and making good use of what we have. It is closely connected to our emotional wellbeing and happiness.

We feel loved and at peace with ourselves for a major part of our lives when we make this attitude ours. This adds and helps us to get rid of greed, amenity, bitterness, jealousy, and promotes a healthy and nurturing attitude towards others, which in turn gets reciprocated and we feel the sense of healthy living. On the face of it we ought to know that a positive and good living is an attitude that makes you feel good about who you are, what you do, and what your potentials are. This attitude impels you to utilize all that you are endowed with as a person, to achieve the highest possible goals. When we have this attitude, we are able to work without any external pressure to perform but there is sufficient pressure and motivation from within.

Positive thinking and a positive attitude of happy life is a joy for ever

The possessing of happy living is like any other habit, so we need to follow the routine of habit formation here as well. You will win new friends and admirers without having to impress them or conform to the pressure of doing things their way. You will be bubbling with life. You will be rearing to go and accomplish all you can with your new found confidence. The best part of adopting the 'positive thinking and a positive attitude of gratitude is that, you will be able to enjoy the smallest pleasures of nature with a heightened sense of satisfaction and awe. We can see and watch a beautiful flower and carry that joy in our mind for future enjoyment with a clear positive habit. We can go back to work freshen and can use it as an object to meditate on when we feel stressed.

When we have this attitude, we are able to work without any external pressure to perform but there is sufficient pressure and motivation from within. The habit of happy living is like any other habit, so we need to follow the routine of habit formation here as well.

LEAVE WORRIES NOW
BE HAPPY ENJOY LIFE
CHAPTER 24

NEGATIVITY TO POSTIVITY

We need to learn a lesson from every situation. No matter how difficult the situation may appear. We should recognize the beautiful lessons waiting to be discovered. Sometimes lessons may prove to be expensive and costly, but every problem is a learning experience in disguise. We need to be conscious of our thoughts, especially, when life just isn't going our way. The moment we see that we are diving into frustration, agony, sorrow or low self –esteem we must shift our thoughts, by thinking about something completely different and unrelated. This will strangle the pattern of self-pity, mind-created imaginations, and negative downward stairs. Really what makes us different from other mammals is our ability to control our thoughts and think for ourselves positively and shift our negative thoughts to a positive angle. We may have made mistakes, but now we can accept it and continue, knowing that we will make a different decision in the future. If we understand this it can be appreciative for the experience. We cannot be both angry and grateful at the same time. We should start counting the blessings and miracles in our lives and if we start exploring for them and we would find more. We should console our mind as to what's not there to be grateful? It's quite true that we are alive and breathing! We have to realize how lucky we are with all the positivity in abundance in our lives. Our mind and body becomes dumb and mum when it comes to pressure, all it wants to do is take the easiest way out and to throw out of us our negative within us.

Feeling good about ourselves and showing self-confidence boosts our skills potential and capabilities in any areas of work and supports us to become more positive. We need to shift our thoughts from being a negative person to more strong a positive man. Also keeping in mind that pushing things to the limit and going beyond what we think is possible for us to get to the next step of being positive. It becomes another key to achieving what we really want to do. Even if it may even be relationships and we are finding it difficult to meet someone where we are actually interested in, we need not wait because it usually doesn't come to us by own, we must stand up to get help from any learned fellow. One of the most important things while doing all of this is to be happy about what we are doing, thus we ought to have a successful goal setting our lifestyle with a positive attitude. At times we may suffer from chronic depression, though we know how good things look on to others life cannot be worse for us. Let's imagine how to deal when life leaves a great big steaming pile at our doorstep. Lest we need to remember that external factors can be dealt with by taking positive steps to repair or at least address the root of the problem as best as we can. Whatever may be the primary cause of the problem, that cause must be examined first?. We may or may not be able to solve the problem, per se, but at least knowing that we are taking positive steps can help us improve our outlook. It will not be easy, of course, for us and it may be like suffering a chronic disease thus we must balance ourselves as "being positive" with an understanding that the reality is, it's going to be an ongoing battle for our own survival. Depression will undermine even the strongest of wills, need help to maintain or at least be reminded of a positive outlook. Counseling, psychotherapy, and the right combination of medication will play a crucial role in helping to keep us from sinking into that very dark place that is the essence of depression.

Be patient, but don't look for miracles. It may be that we
will need the help of professionals throughout our lives to
maintain a generally even keel. If one could "will away"
depression, there would be no need of doctors or drugs.
What we can do is understand why we feel like we do, and
explain to our counselors that we wish it were that easy,
and that we appreciate our concern towards positivity.
Shifting our thoughts enables us to the right path of our
positivity and thinking in its direction of positivity can
make us to lead a very happy life. What is required is that
we never wanted to see the good in ourselves and,
therefore, didn't want to see it in others also. We must not
be critical and condescending rather we must be
encouraging and supportive. We should not try to treat
others as we would like to be treated, but also try to
consider how we would like to be treated. The world likes
to appreciate positivity, and the more we share it with
others, the more we would be practicing it your own lives.
When we start feeling like the idea of not being a positive
person we need to remind ourselves that all it takes is one
tiny step in the right direction to move towards a more
positive attitude. We have to believe in ourselves and
remember the most important lesson of all is a positive
outlook and that is a choice that we can always make. The
power of remaining positive, whatever the situation, can
never be underestimated. We are all here for a short
duration, but is it worth it to spend any of that time in a any
angry or being negative? That need to sort out in mind and
soul and thus must share our positive thoughts with others.
The real test of any one is to remain positive whenever
some challenges become difficult. Remaining positive
keeps our mind in the right state of balance and often opens
resolutions to the problems at hand. Negativity is
contagious and spreads like fire. It not only does its affect
anyone, but it spreads to everyone who ever comes in
contact with it or whoever they interact with.

When only the negative perspective is in focus, the resolution process is impeded. Eliminating negativity, or rather, being positive is a mindset that can be found at any moment, and which can be turned into a habit. We must throw away the negativity in us and opt for being a very positive person. What is Positive Thinking? The feeling of positivity within us. It is said that positive thinking is purely an internal matter. It has nothing to do with our external circumstances. There is something positive within us which helps us to keep us happy and there is something negative within us which makes us unhappy. Happy living through positivity is nothing more than living a normal life free from undue pressures, problems and tensions. If we want to live a happy life then we need to get rid of the negativity within us and above all we must start thinking positive which will not make us unhappy. Negative thinking always complicates the problems and increases unhappiness. Most of us do the mistake of looking outwards for happiness rather than looking inward. Think positive, be strong, be bold and be courageous every day. Even if we are having a bad day, think of some good things that may come our way, either later that day, tomorrow, next hour, month, or year. When everything seems to be beyond our control, it's almost too easy for us to slip into the grasp of negativity. To avoid negativity we must strive to abolish this sort of thinking through the power of thinking positively. The art of positive thinking is not a complicated kind of art difficult to learn rather a simple art of positive thinking, like eating well, living well and feeling well. What we need to do is just to tune up our mind to enjoy every moment of life and let the positive thinking follow us. This is something that needs to be looked into thoroughly. We need to focus on the positive aspects rather than on the negative setbacks. We must remember that good and happy living is the reward of positive thinking.

We ought to remember, only positive thinking can bring happiness in our lives. If we cannot think positively, we cannot live happily. Being our own teacher or adviser we ought to look everything with a positive angle. Let us find something good even in most critical moments of our life and let us make positive thinking the basis of our happy living. It's a matter of thought that fools worry about the circumstances on which they have no control. Why worry when we cannot change anything or the climate, rather enjoy it whether it's hot, humid, cold, cloudy, foggy and snowy. Let us all keep our mind body and soul pleasant all the time. A sound and positive happiness is all around. It's not far away from us. If we do not want to live happy, it's up to us. It's our own choice. We must not blame others, nor should we blame our fate or external circumstances. Another thing is that feeling confident affects the way we perceive our situations and how we decide to manage them. Think that by being more optimistic we alter our approaches to situations and take on them in a healthier manner; we think of alternatives and act according to better outcomes. If we think positive it will be positive. It does not say to stick our heads in the soil; rather it says to think positive. Interestingly it does not say feel positive it says think positive and that is the real meaning to remain happy. Happiness does not come alone, it adds our mind body and soul to remain in constant touch with each other. We have to remove negative thoughts and create and atmosphere to be happy in our lives. There are many fear factors that are reasoning us to be unhappy and the main reason being that our heart and our feelings which are more susceptible to fear and worry then the mind. Of course we do the worrying in our minds but it is our emotions that are worried not our brains. When the heart senses the possibility of loss it can start panicking and then uses the mind to worry and many times tries to manipulate the brain in dealing with the fear.

The heart desires something and gets excited about it and then it manipulates the mind to assure that it will get it. Although the brain can control the emotions and knowledge precedes all, however when it comes to response time the brain is slower than the emotions. That is which explains why we say or do things and then regret them. Our objective in life should be to train ourselves to wait for the brain to show up before we say or do anything. Fear usually comes from the emotions and thinking positive is something the brain is capable of doing. So always think positive. It would be very hard to tell someone who is worried to be good and happy by feeling positive. But if you tell them to think positive that is something even a worried person can do. We need to use our mind to think positive, to think of a positive outcome. Thinking positive brings positive results in its wake; when you react in a positive way to a negative situation you usually get positive in return. Positive mental attitude is effective in many ways. There are limits to the effectiveness of positive thinking. It is not always enough to change deeply entrenched irrational core beliefs about self, others and the world. When someone does something to us do we think about it in a positive way or in a negative way? Do we try to assume that the person who is not treating us the way we should be treated is themselves in pain and needs our love or do we assume that they just don't like us and therefore we need to respond back in kind? It is therefore a must for us to learn understand and remember that we need to be positive and think positive in the interest of our good happy living.

LEAVE WORRIES NOW
BE HAPPY ENJOY LIFE

CHAPTER 25

WHY NOT LIVE HAPPILY AND SWEETLY

Thought which are provoking our mind, about the uncertainties and the negativities, as to what will happen tomorrow. Worries that are prevailing in our minds are repetitive thoughts associated with feelings of anxiety in anticipation of some negative future event. Whether the worries are about financial crisis, family problems, work, health or any topic of concern, the anxious feelings produced and sustained by the imaginary thoughts which always distinctly appear to be unpleasant. Positive

Thinking leads us to a happy life one must not forgot the life is what we make it, so let us make it a happy one! Don't worry on things that may not happen, life is too short to worry too much. Smile and be happy. Make yourself to be positive person. Keep smiling in the sunlight. Imagine every day to be a positive day and the last of a life surrounded with hopes, the hours that come unexpectedly will be much the more grateful.

The mind that is anxious about future events is miserable. Present fears are less than horrible imaginings. Positive thinking is sure to ward of every odd imagination and sure to make you a happy person. Happy living actually means approaching life's challenges with a positive outlook.

It does not necessarily mean avoiding or ignoring the bad things; instead, it involves making the most of potentially bad situations, trying to see the best in other people, and viewing yourself and your abilities in a positive light. Happy living centers on such things as a belief in abilities, a positive approach to challenges, and trying to make the most of bad situations. Bad things will happen. Sometimes you will be disappointed or hurt by the actions of others. This does not mean that the world is out to get you or that all people will let you down. Instead, happy living will look at the situation realistically, search for ways that they can improve the situation, and try to learn from their experiences. Happy living brings good cheer, remembering that the misfortunes hardest to bear are those that never happen, focus on the positive aspects of lives, rather than on the negative setbacks. Let us not waste our lives in doubts and fears. It is not work that kills us, it is worry and the negative thinking. Work is healthy; but worry is rust upon the blade. It is not movement that destroys the machinery, but friction. We need to forget the most disturbing negative thinking in our lives and opt for the positive attitude by following the principles of happy living. Not only can happy living impact our ability to cope with stress and our immunity, it also has an impact on our overall well-being. Our success lies only in our happy living. Look to be happy think in positive terms and think as if the unhappiness is not there at lot and God has given us this precious life to enjoy to our fullest all the fruits of happiness of our lives. Happy living and good living is definitely an "Art of Sweet Living".

CREATE HAPPINESS WITHIN YOU

If you are interested in getting more happiness, to get it through positive thinking. all you need to do is to focus on all the directions on positive thinking as if you have already attained success. You need to focus on the thing and create a life within you. If you want love and affection, entertain people and give them the abundance of love. If you want to have greater health, pay attention on all the ways that make us healthy, thus creating and delivering a good life within you by thinking in positive ways. You need to understand and admit that there are problems that you cannot change. But you can change the ways of your thinking if you identify the main reason of the problem. And if you acknowledge the facts, that you have been negative or inactive in finding a solution to the problem, probably this will make it easier for you to become positive thus creating a new lease of life within you. Positive thinking will surely make you happy. Another thing to understand is that you must try to make goals. Making goals can give you a more positive outlook on life. People often tend to get bored with life and get the feeling that they are stuck to negative things with the result they often get the feeling of being depressed dejected and monotonous. Setting a direction and a goal for yourself, would surely help you to move forward. If you are expecting to succeed, and are not afraid of failure, you have the best chance of staying positive and can create a very positive life within you. When you, or any of your associates, are tempted to worry about a problem, write out the solution and a definite answer to it. This helps a positive feeling to generate within you.

The perfect way to conquer worry is the Prayer of God

Another thing you need to understand is that there are several ways to cultivate a mental attitude that can bring you peace and happiness and can carnage a good life within you. More of it if you fill your mind with thoughts of peace, courage, health, and hope, your life will be easy to live. If you think in positive terms you would get a happy feeling of life and mind you if you let yourself to forget your own unhappiness, by trying to create a little happiness for others you are sure to get happiness in your live. You are best to yourself. The perfect way to conquer worry is the Prayer of God. To keep yourself from worrying about criticism, do not even try to get mixed with your enemies, because if you do you will hurt yourself far more than we hurting them. You will fall prey to negative thinking and this in turn will lead you unhappiness in life. Instead of worrying about ingratitude, let's expect it. Let's remember that the only way to find happiness is not to expect gratitude, but to give for the joy of giving. Let us build a happy life within us generate peace and a healthy atmosphere around us. This will help us to lead a peaceful happy and prosperous life and we would find ourselves to be happier than before. You should do things in the order of their importance. If you have or face problems in hand you need to clear your desk of all papers except those relating to the immediate problem at hand. When you face a problem, solve it then and there, by thinking positively and if you have the facts to make a decision, make a decision fast and do not linger on. Learn to think in positive terms organize the things, deputize, and supervise straight away by coming to decision.

Simply postponing it would spoil your good thoughts and there is every likelihood your mind may get into negative activities and start thinking in negative manner. Therefore think positive, write down a list of things that make you positive, however big, small, likely or unlikely. Then work to make them occur more often. Look for moments of joy and savor them. Recognize your good happening every day. Be positive think positive and be happy.

Take care of your health- Eat Well

One need not to forgot that we need to eat well do plenty of exercise and do not skip meals It is a known fact that physical exercise is known to stimulate our veins and get to strengthen our minds that lift depression and anxiety, so we need to walk, swim, run or whatever we like doing best above all we must move ahead in direction where our mind can generate electricity to think in positive direct. So take care of your health and eat well. Those who create negativity or those who not well tend to give themselves worry and stress and in the end tend to be devastated. If we cannot get some good sunshine, we can always lighten up our thoughts with brighter lights of positive thinking. We can have ample of lunch of positive thinking. To avoid negative thoughts we need to take frequent walks No man is indispensable and no man is not capable of positive thinking. Our friends are always there to give us some moral support. Spending time and engaging ourselves in worthwhile positive activities could give us a very enjoyable and satisfying feeling. Nothing feels better than having group support and talking in terms of positive thinking.

Good friends are quite important and their company generally lightened up our spirits. This makes us to think in positive manner and to get to know such friends we simply have to be friendly with ourselves, and then the friendships will naturally follow us and make our lives happy. We need to understand the power of positive thinking and its support and we have not to underestimate it strength and support. Don't we feel so good when someone pats us on our back and gives us some words of encouragement during your most challenging times and difficult times and advises us to remain positive and think positive just hug or embrace someone with positive attitude someday you will see that you have almost changed his life. Get intimate with him and try to establish close ties with his family and friends. The love and care expressed by you will tremendously boost him in positive manner and well as your immune system and fury of worry will be diminished for all if you advise them to think in positive terms. In our lives difficulties and storms may come and go in the form of reversals, but if we have the power of positive thinking and foundation of inner fulfillment we would be able to deal with it with a very clear practical mind and with this positive thinking these storms will not kill us nor will disrupt us. There could be numberless reasons for which we keep on worrying. We may be worried about our health, wealth, loved ones, friends, the happening of yesterday and the follow happenings of tomorrow, the environment or the world politics, but these can be dealt with firm mind and fearless worry if we generate within ourselves the power of positive thinking within ourselves.

LEAVE WORRIES NOW
BE HAPPY ENJOY LIFE
CHAPTER 26

START HAPPY LIVING

Even when you are facing challenges, it is important to stay open to laughter and humor. Sometimes, simply recognizing the potential humor in a situation can lessen your stress and brighten your outlook. Seeking out sources of humor such as watching a funny sitcom or reading jokes online can help you think more positive thoughts. We need to know and realize that nobody is perfect or flawless. If we try to change the way we look, talk and behave just to please others, and show our pride we will gradually become such a person that we ourselves won't recognize each other and would start and create unnecessary worries within us and our surrounding without being positive and will not start to live happily. We ought to stop worrying over unnecessary things be positive and live without fear happily. As a result, negative thoughts can creep into your mind. While you know that thinking positively is better for your state of mind, you might be surprised to learn that it can also be good for your health. We need to understand that what people think of us is their concern, and not ours. If they think about us to be, too reticent or proud, it's really not our business. If every time we happen to meet some new fellows, we may wonder and imagine as what they think of us, and with this feeling in us we will never be able to live a trouble-free and hassle free life. We are bound to fall into the trap of unnecessary worries denying us the startup of new and the happy living life. We must think rationally. Is it in our hands or can we control what others think about us? Simply we need to ignore them.

If we cannot, and live our lives the way we want to and find the ways to leave worries aside and start living a happy life. Let us make our way to happy living.

Positive Thinking with Positive Attitudes.

Positive thinking is not about putting on a pair of rose-colored glasses and ignoring all the negative things you will encounter in life. That approach can be just as devastating as ignoring the positive and only focusing on the negative. Balance, with a healthy dose of realism, is the key. It is a well-known fact that attitude decides how a natives or persons copes up with the day to day events of life. Attitude is what a influence a person's reaction to a situation in life is. It sets the emotional undertone for a person to his likes or dislikes a situation even before he is acquainted with it. Positive attitude is a quality that is second to none in a human being. Though we attach so much importance to this attitude, as we grow into teenage and adult years we find ourselves becoming ungrateful or taking things for granted. We lose touch with the very same qualities that we instill in our children. We take for granted our life, our health, our families, the people in our lives, the things that our loved ones do for us to make our lives easier and things that we possess. The attitude of positive speaks a lot about a person. It denotes about changing negative attitudes and making positive thinking a positive attitude a good habit. Thinking positively and a positive attitude help us to appreciate and value ourselves, our potential and all that we have. It ensures that we do not take our abilities for granted. It makes us look at ourselves as special people with a special set of abilities and potential. It banishes the feelings of inadequacy and insecurity that arises from unfair comparisons with others.

It helps us to appreciate people for who they are and not magnify what they are not and their little flaws. It drives away prejudice and makes us approach life with an open mind. It predisposes us to react to the daily events of life in a positive manner and help us to look at the brighter side of life. Make us optimistic. It gives hope and helps us look forward to life with anticipation. We need to know that positive thinking takes the focus away from what we don't have, to appreciating and making good use of what we have. It is closely connected to our emotional wellbeing and happiness. We feel loved and at peace with ourselves for a major part of our lives when we make this attitude ours. This adds and helps us to get rid of greed, amenity, bitterness, jealousy, and promotes a healthy and nurturing attitude towards others, which in turn gets reciprocated and we feel the sense of healthy living. We attach so much importance to this attitude of gratitude that when our children fail to thank someone, we insist that they do it. That is what is needed to be avoided from time to time. We expect this in return from others when we help them or give them a gift. We call a person discourteous and rude when they do not say thank us in return. On the face of it we ought to know that a positive is not an attitude of being satisfied and content, that you never want to do anything, anymore. This is an attitude that makes you feel good about who you are, what you do, and what your potentials are. This attitude impels you to utilize all that you are endowed with as a person, to achieve the highest possible goals. When we have this attitude, we are able to work without any external pressure to perform but there is sufficient pressure and motivation from within. The possessing of positive thinking is like any other habit, so we need to follow the routine of habit formation here as well. You will win new friends and admirers without having to impress them or conform to the pressure of doing things their way. You will be bubbling with life and the joie de vivre.

You will be rearing to go and accomplish all you can with your new found confidence. The best part of adopting the 'positive thinking and a positive attitude of gratitude is that, you will be able to enjoy the smallest pleasures of nature with a heightened sense of satisfaction and awe. I can see and watch a beautiful flower and carry that joy in my mind for future enjoyment with a clear positive habit. I can go back to work freshen and can use it as an object to meditate on when I feel stressed. Let us be clear that a positive is not an attitude of being satisfied and content, that you never want to do anything, anymore. This is an attitude that makes you feel good about who you are, what you do, and what your potentials are. This attitude impels you to utilize all that you are endowed with as a person, to achieve the highest possible goals. When we have this attitude, we are able to work without any external pressure to perform but there is sufficient pressure and motivation from within. The habit of positive thinking is like any other habit, so we need to follow the routine of habit formation here as well.

LEAVE WORRIES NOW
BE HAPPY ENJOY LIFE
CHAPTER 27

ALWAYS THINK POSITVE - FORGET WORRIES

Being a positive thinker is not about ignoring reality in favor of aspirational thoughts. It is more about taking a proactive approach to your life. Instead of feeling hopeless or overwhelmed, positive thinking allows you to tackle life's challenges by looking for effective ways to resolve conflict and come up with creative solutions to problems. It might not be easy, but the positive impact it will have on your mental, emotional, and physical health will be well-worth it. At time we may think that there is no road is left for us from where we can achieve the happiness of our lives. We may also feel that life has become terrible for us to live and we are carrying new hope that someone would come to rescue us. There may be chances that someone who was there with us before might have held on to us when we were on the dark side of the life.

What if when everything goes wrong and all the doors of happiness are closed our live becomes a silent. It is a quite common and we are aware of a marvelous proverb that Life itself is a stage and we all are the performers, performing different acts assigned to us by our almighty power. We should not forget as to what is in our possession?, if it is to fulfill our duties towards our responsibility and do whatever is correct and is allowed by us in our life? We should not forget that happiness in life comes through the doors of positive thoughts; we need to have them first. If one door happen to close, another opens, in the event only when we are confident and optimistic.

We have so many reasons to cry and at the same time plenty of reasons to smile as well. Similarly, happiness does not stand for anything, but is on our way of thinking that how do we keep ourselves happy in life. Failure and disappointment are part of our life. The only thing is that we need to face and solve the problem is by keeping our dreams and hope alive be it a reason that success and happiness will come our way again. There are quite a number of reasons to believe that for a successful and happy life the mystery surrounding it lies in our interests, and good memory which is the basis of our interest, power of desire and aim, keeping ourselves smiling and the doubt free character which is the foremost important reason for a successful and happy life. If we possess one solid unselfish and doubt free character within ourselves we would be quite happy and successful. The experience has taught us that we should buy some strength, hope and positivity from our loved ones to help ourselves in such a situation rather than surrendering as life is a precious gift of God and is equipped with full of joy and happiness if we help ourselves in these critical moments we can live with considerable optimism.

Now let's us imagine that we are not feeling at our best today, and we are having thoughts that could be classified as negative. We shouldn't be thinking such negative thoughts. We don't like the negative thoughts. We ought to know that negative thoughts are stressful, demoralizing and depressing. We shouldn't aim to have negative thoughts at all. Often we feel uncomfortable because we think we have to say or do something in response to another person's words. When we find ourselves thinking this way, it helps enormously to take a few moments to check inside and notice what we are feeling. We are deeply depressed that negativity has governed us and has taken a deep root in our minds.

So, let's imagine that you have chosen to focus on your negative thinking with regards to school. The next step is to spend a little bit of time each day evaluating your own thoughts. When you find yourself thinking critical thoughts about yourself, take a moment to pause and reflect. While you might be upset about getting a bad grade on an exam, is berating yourself really the best approach? Is there any way to put a positive spin on the situation? While you might not have done well on this exam, at least you have a better indication of how to structure your study time for the next big test. However, despite of all these good thoughts which are embodied to us by the almighty fail to revive these unwanted circumstances that lead us to sorrow and difficulties and a situation where we do not know what is correct and good for us and what is wrong for us. We should always remember that, "Life is there, where there is hope". That single thing that remains in our hands is to find out ways to know how to overcome these worries of our life at that very moment when all doors are closed for us which means that whatever situation is there, we must not give up hope. We must fight because there have been always a chance that with good faith and hard work we can turn the odds in our favor. It is often said that it is very easy to advice but when it comes to us, things go out of our control and we fail to suggest a way out for ourselves. We fall into the trap of unnecessary worries and elope ourselves with negative thoughts. We feel better when somebody else is facing some difficulty but when it comes to us we fail to gather that faith, will power and the words of strength. Being a positive thinker is not about ignoring reality in favor of aspirational thoughts. It is more about taking a proactive approach to your life. Instead of feeling hopeless or overwhelmed, positive thinking allows you to tackle life's challenges by looking for effective ways to resolve conflict and come up with creative solutions to problems.

It might not be easy, but the positive impact it will have on your mental, emotional, and physical health will be well-worth it. It takes practice; lots of practice. This is not a step-by-step process that you can complete and be done with. Instead, it involves a lifelong commitment to looking inside yourself and being willing to challenge negative thoughts and make positive changes.It is a common fact that no one in this world is free of obstacles or difficulties. If all the openings of happiness are shut for us and we have to overcome that and have no way to come out, but to survive lest we must have to learn to swim out of the sorrows because this is what is called life and sorrow free living. There are lot more examples and in many other situations, where we will find that how we could have faced and fought with our sorrows and difficulties of life when there was no hope left in our lives. When the power of will is at the worst and each one of us knows that the one who is gone never comes back. Neither a thousands of words would not be enough to bring him back nor a million tears, because each and every moment, eyes would only shed tears , mind would remain tensed and we would be simply surrounded by worries and the life seems to have been vanished. Life is ever expanding, contraction is death. As commonly said by big saints that the self- seeking man who is looking after his personal comforts and leading a lazy life for himself there would be no room for him even in the hell and he simply have lost the power of his will. One cannot do anything without it. We fail only when we do not try very hard to achieve the power and faith within us. As soon as we lose faith, death comes in our way and we are surrounds by all the evils and stupid worries of the world. The secret and history of every successful man is to have, good confidence, faith and strength behind him and that remain the right cause of his single success in life. Unselfishness plays a very vital role in his life.

He may not have been perfectly unselfish, yet he was tending towards it. If he had been perfectly unselfish, he would have been as great a success. The degree of unselfishness marks the degree of success everywhere and he leads to be successful man without fear worries and selfishness. Therefore creation of positivity in life is utmost necessary to enjoy the special gift of God to us. The love for God and worshipping God adds to one common thing the immense faith in Him. There may be different beliefs and ways to worship God in different communities, places and religions, but one thing remains the same and that is the Love of God for all of us. Our world is full of odds and evens, happiness and sorrows, fulfilment and emptiness. And these are all created by the Almighty. However, the most beautiful Gift of God, is Human, which is such a mystery driven by Him which could hardly be defined or explained in depth. We know that life cannot be foreseen. Life is not a bed of roses. Life is a battle field and not a bed of roses as every man on earth has to struggle very hard in making his life happy. If aim of our life is to stay happy and let others to be happy, we will be happy and remembered by all. But no one will actually remember us for the wealth we have gained, or success we have achieved. I have no aim in life. Summary living with no purpose in life is just like a feather moving towards the wind. Life is such a special gift of Almighty and it is not gifted by Him to use it the way we like or love to. The actual path shown by Him needs to be followed by us for us to reach the peak of betterment every moment. We need to have some positive attitude to look at it comfortably but at the same time having a positive mental attitude does not mean banishing all negative thoughts and people from your life. One and another one arises. Change your attitude from negative thinking to Positive Thinking and converge yourself from negativity to positivity.

Positive thinking is a mental and emotional attitude that focuses on the bright side of life and expects positive results. A positive person anticipates happiness, health and success, and believes he or she can overcome any obstacle and difficulty. Positive thinking is not accepted by everyone. Some, consider it as nonsense, and scoff at people who follow it, but there is a growing number of people, who accept positive thinking as a fact, and believe in its effectiveness. We need to learn a lesson from every situation. No matter how difficult the situation may appear. We should recognize the beautiful lessons waiting to be discovered. Sometimes lessons may prove to be expensive and costly, but every problem is a learning experience in disguise. We need to be conscious of our thoughts, especially, when life just isn't going our way. The moment we see that we are diving into frustration, agony, sorrow or low self –esteem we must shift our thoughts, by thinking about something completely different and unrelated.

Negative thinking is contagious.

We affect, and are affected by the people we meet, in one way or another. This happens instinctively and on a subconscious level, through words, thoughts and feelings, and through body language. Is it any wonder that we want to be around positive people, and prefer to avoid negative ones? People are more disposed to help us, if we are positive, and they dislike and avoid anyone broadcasting negativity. Negative thoughts, words and attitude, create negative and unhappy feelings, moods and behavior. When the mind is negative, poisons are released into the blood, which cause more unhappiness and negativity. This is the way to failure, frustration and disappointment. Individuals with a pessimistic explanatory style often blame themselves when bad things happen, but fail to give themselves adequate credit for successful outcomes.

They also have a tendency to view negative events as expected and lasting. As you can imagine, blaming yourself for events outside of your control or viewing these unfortunate events as a persistent part of your life can have a detrimental impact on your state of mind. Positive thinkers are more apt to use an optimistic explanatory style, but the way in which people attribute events can also vary depending upon the exact situation. This will strangle the pattern of self-pity, mind-created imaginations, and negative downward stairs. Really what makes us different from other mammals is our ability to control our thoughts and think for ourselves positively and shift our negative thoughts to a positive angle. We may have made mistakes, but now we can accept it and continue, knowing that we will make a different decision in the future. If we understand this it can be appreciative for the experience. We cannot be both angry and grateful at the same time. We should start counting the blessings and miracles in our lives and if we start exploring for them and we would find more. It's quite true that we are alive and breathing! We have to realize how lucky we are with all the positivity in abundance in our lives. Our mind and body becomes dumb and mum when it comes to pressure, all it wants to do is take the easiest way out and to throw out of us our negative within us. While the terms positive thinking and positive psychology are sometimes used interchangeably, it is important to understand that they are not the same thing. First, positive thinking is about looking at things from a positive point of view. Positive psychology certainly tends to focus on optimism, but it also notes that while there are many benefits to thinking positively, there are actually times when more realistic thinking is more advantageous. Feeling good about ourselves and showing self-confidence boosts our skills potential and capabilities in any areas of work and supports us to become more positive.

We need to shift our thoughts from being a negative person to more strong a positive man. Also keeping in mind that pushing things to the limit and going beyond what we think is possible for us to get to the next step of being positive. It becomes another key to achieving what we really want to do. You have probably had someone tell you to "look on the bright side" or to "see the cup as half full." Chances are good that the people who make these comments are positive thinkers. Even if it may even be relationships and we are finding it difficult to meet someone where we are actually interested in, we need not wait because it usually doesn't come to us by own, we must stand up to get help from any learned fellow. One of the most important things while doing all of this is to be happy about what we are doing, thus we ought to have a successful goal setting our lifestyle with a positive attitude. At times we may suffer from chronic depression, though we know how good things look on to others life cannot be worse for us. Let's imagine how to deal when life leaves a great big steaming pile at our doorstep. Lest we need to remember that external factors can be dealt with by taking positive steps to repair or at least address the root of the problem as best as we can. Whatever may be the primary cause of the problem, that cause must be examined first? We may or may not be able to solve the problem, per se, but at least knowing that we are taking positive steps can help us improve our outlook. It will not be easy, of course, for us and it may be like suffering a chronic disease thus we must balance ourselves as "being positive" with an understanding that the reality is, it's going to be an ongoing battle for our own survival. Depression will undermine even the strongest of wills, need help to maintain or at least be reminded of a positive outlook. Counseling, psychotherapy, and the right combination of medication will play a crucial role in helping to keep us from sinking into that very dark place that is the essence of depression.

Be patient, but don't look for miracles. It may be that we will need the help of professionals throughout our lives to maintain a generally even keel. If one could "will away" depression, there would be no need of doctors or drugs. What we can do is understand why we feel like we do, and explain to our counselors that we wish it were that easy, and that we appreciate our concern towards positivity. Shifting our thoughts enables us to the right path of our positivity and thinking in its direction of positivity can make us to lead a very happy life.

FORGET NEGATIVE THINKING

Never let life's hardships disturb you .no one can avoid problems, not even saints or sages. As with any habit, the habit of remaining positive in all situations takes practice and a commitment to yourself to take control. If you tend to think positive you stand to gain all the amenities of a happy life. Positive Thinking leads you to a happy life one must not forgot the life is what you make it, so make it a happy one! Don't worry on things that may not happen, life is too short to worry too much. Smile and be happy. Make yourself to be positive person. Don't hold onto anything that bothers your mind. It can only hurt your health and it won't help your problems at all. The people that live the longest in this world do not hold grudges or hold or fall prey into negative feelings. Visualize your worries on a large chalkboard in your mind. Watch yourself take a big eraser and erase the problems. Every time the thoughts come back into your head, see yourself with the eraser again. Keep your slate clean and form a habit of thinking positive. We must not worry about tomorrow, for tomorrow will worry about itself. Each day has enough trouble of its own. Do not anticipate trouble, or worry about what may never happen.

Keep in the sunlight. Imagine every day to be a positive day and the last of a life surrounded with hopes, the hours that come unexpectedly will be much the more grateful. The mind that is anxious about future events is miserable. Present fears are less than horrible imaginings. Positive thinking is sure to ward of every odd imagination and sure to make you a happy person. Positive thinking actually means approaching life's challenges with a positive outlook. It does not necessarily mean avoiding or ignoring the bad things; instead, it involves making the most of potentially bad situations, trying to see the best in other people, and viewing yourself and your abilities in a positive light. Positive thinking centers on such things as a belief in your abilities, a positive approach to challenges, and trying to make the most of bad situations. Bad things will happen. Sometimes you will be disappointed or hurt by the actions of others. This does not mean that the world is out to get you or that all people will let you down. Instead, positive thinkers will look at the situation realistically, search for ways that they can improve the situation, and try to learn from their experiences. Positive attitude bring good cheer, remembering that the misfortunes hardest to bear are those that never happen, focus on the positive aspects of lives, rather than on the negative setbacks. Let us not waste our lives in doubts and fears. It is not work that kills us, it is worry and the negative thinking. Work is healthy; but worry is rust upon the blade. It is not movement that destroys the machinery, but friction. We need to forget the most disturbing negative thinking in our lives and opt for the positive attitude by following the principles of positive thinking. Not only can positive thinking impact your ability to cope with stress and your immunity, it also has an impact on your overall well-being.

LEAVE WORRIES NOW
BE HAPPY ENJOY LIFE

CHAPTER 28

ANALYZING POSITIVITY

Thought which are provoking our mind, about the uncertainties and the negativities, as to what will happen tomorrow. Worries that are prevailing in our minds are repetitive thoughts associated with feelings of anxiety in anticipation of some negative future event. Whether the worries are about financial crisis, family problems, work, health or any topic of concern, the anxious feelings produced and sustained by the imaginary thoughts which always distinctly appear to be unpleasant. Worrying will carry tomorrow's load with today's strength. Worry will not empty tomorrow of its sorrows, it empties today of its power and strength. Worries make you to move into tomorrow ahead of time. Half the worry in the world is caused by people trying to make decisions before they have sufficient knowledge on which to base a decision. Why worry about the future. Just imagine as to what if we just acted like everything was easy and there was nothing very serious about it to come in future. Worry often gives a small thing a big shadow and its surrounding do frightened with more scary things. Why worry about tomorrow; concentrate on today happening as for tomorrow will worry about itself. Each day has its own worries and troubles. If there is not any solution to the some problem then do not waste time worrying about it. And if there is a solution to the problem then why waste time worrying about it.

Worry will never rob tomorrow of its sorrows, but will only deny today of its meaning happiness and joys. Worrying is actually a form of superstition and creates false images in our mind and that is the main reason and cause which makes and leads us to this point of imagination. A human being can survive almost anything, as long as he or she sees the end in sight. If something bad or good is to happen it is sure to happen, whether we worry or not. Let us put our energy into today and stop worrying about the future and past. We should not foresee trouble, or worry about what may never happen as past is dead and gone forever and future is uncertain and yet to come. The basic facts we should know about worry. The basic techniques to analyze worry and how to break the worry habit before it breaks us. These are the simple ways where we can concentrate and get rid of worries prevailing in our thoughts. Annalise worry to see and get the reasons and facts of worry. To avoid reoccurrence of worries, concentrate on prayers as prayers are the best source of remedies of the prevailing worries. The more you pray, the less you'll panic. The more you worship, the less you worry. There is nothing that wastes the body like worry, and anyone who has any faith in God should need not to worry about anything whatsoever is to happen in future. We ought to know the basic fundamental of analyzing worries. Worries create unnecessary thoughts and these are caused by people going in for unwanted decisions, fore hand not even knowing as to when a good decision is made and not even having sufficient knowledge about it. We must first study and after carefully weighing all the facts than only come to a powerful decision.

Simply making castles in the air won't solve our problems but add more to our vows. Anxiety and worry can go hand in hand. When anxiety grabs the mind, it is self-perpetuating. Your mind gets clogged with numerous with buts and ifs. Do not worry about your life. Worries are repetitive thoughts associated with feelings of anxiety in anticipation of some negative future event. Yet anxious feelings and the worries that lead to them can prove helpful. It becomes a difficult problem if you are constantly anxious as it will become a hindrance to your everyday life, rather than motivate you to some good and better things. Never worry alone. Worrisome thoughts reproduce faster so one of the most powerful ways to stop the spiral of worry is simply to disclose the worry to a friend. What you will eat or drink; or about your body, what you will wear. If you know that the circumstance is beyond your control or power change than revise it to your liking. Just try to put a stop-less order on your worries. Don't permit little things which become insects of life to ruin your happiness. Co-operate with the inevitable. Decide just how much anxiety a thing may be worth and refuse to give in anymore. All the happiness is not given in one go it comes slowly and slowly. If your worries center on, an important relationship in your life, pay special attention to remain positive and be happy. To keep yourself happy, treat your worried thoughts as valuable signals. How to keep from worrying about criticism? Simply unjust criticism is often a disguised compliment. It often means that you have aroused jealousy and envy. Let's keep a record of the fool things we have done and criticize ourselves.

The utmost cause of worry is your state of depression. Worries are there to motivate information-gathering and problem-solving. Depression is the inability to construct a future. Depression is inertia. That's the thing about depression: But depression is so insidious, and it compounds daily, that it's impossible to ever see the end. Depressed people think they know themselves, but maybe they only know depression. There are no hopeless than this to get depressed. Our attitude towards suffering and depression becomes very important because it can affect how we cope with suffering when it arises. Depression is nourished by a lifetime of un grieved and unforgiven causes. Never worry about your heart till it stops beating. How can you deal with anxiety? You might try what when you did. A person worried so much that he decided to hire someone to do his worrying for him. Times will change for the better when you change. Worry is a misuse of the imagination. Worry is most often a prideful way of thinking that you have more control over life and its circumstances than you actually do. To keep yourself happy, treat your worried thoughts as valuable signals. These are the fundamental facts you should be familiar about worries.

A huge factor to stay happy is to cater your worries around, an important relationship in your life and pay special attention sustaining positive relationships. Worries are there to motivate information gathering and problem-solving. Make your mind firm and do come to a positive decision as come what we will not allow the worries to entire our mind and soul.

Once a decision is carefully reached we should get busy carrying out our decisions and should not bother about all the anxieties that are about to come. When we, or any of our colleagues or associates, are about to worry about a problem, we must write it out and think of the following questions: Instead of worrying about what people say of you, why not spend time trying to accomplish something they will admire. What if we just acted like everything was easy? How would your life be different if you stopped worrying about things we can't control and started focusing on the things we can? Let today be the day. You free yourself from fruitless worry, seize the day and take effective action on things you can change.

LEAVE WORRIES NOW
BE HAPPY ENJOY LIFE
CHAPTER 29

WHAT DO YOU GET OUT OF BEING NEGATIVE?

You may feel largely uncomfortable, when worries attack your thoughts and mind which makes worrying about a situation an easier option to get depressed and diffused. While you are consuming more worries you are far too busy to do anything else to fix the real problem and would rather find it hard to get into a smart solution. Thus resulting in a fact that you spend your evenings worrying only without even bothering to find some time to search a new job. You get nothing out of worrying except only to think and cry. Another cause of getting worried is the attachment with which your inner soul gets attracted to. Attachment brings worry. If you have a problem and you come up with the answer, you stop worrying immediately. Our minds can be dishonest, persuading us that we are worrying about something, when our deepest fear is entirely different. No-one likes to admit that they've chosen to worry. The first step is to write down your worries, which will help you make sense of them, and then decide on one small step you can take towards a solution. But to be very true no man in this world is free of obstacles or difficulties. Don't make worry your habit. Break this habit and stop all the negative and panic thoughts provoking your mind all the time. If you can't change the past, but you must not ruin the present by worrying about the future.

Joy is what happens to us when we allow ourselves to recognize how good things really are. When we feel worried and depressed, we need to consciously form a smile on our faces and act upbeat until the happy feeling becomes genuine reality. Feelings of depression and hopelessness and or anger are even tougher to cope with on a consistent basis. When you are worried, you not only hurt yourself, but the limited support systems that are still holding on your mind but making you to get more and more worried and nothing is achieved in terms of success except the re-carnation of worries and worries.......

Your actions breed confidence and courage. If you want to conquer fear, anger and worry do not sit ideal and just think about it. Let our deep worrying become advance thinking and planning. If you look into your own mind and heart, and you find nothing wrong there, what is there to worry about? Practically nothing what is there to fear about and again nothing? So why worry unnecessarily and make your present and future dark. Why being a negative person and what do you get out of it being a depression dejected and sad man.? Why not turn your thoughts to be a positive person simply it is a question of tilting your mind towards a positive side of thing. See both the aspects of a situation and ways the pros and cons of both the sides and try to abolish the negativity in you. Think of the best the best is sure to happen and if you think of the worst the worst will come. Better come forward wake up and think positive first. Positive persons always succeed in life whatever be the circumstances and the negative often dig a death trap for themselves. So why be a negative person why you have all the qualities of being a positive man.

If you are interested in getting more happiness, focus on all the ways as if you have already attained success. You need to focus on the thing and create a live within you. If you want love and affection, focus on all the people and the abundance of love that you have to give to them. If we want to have greater health, focus on all the ways that we are healthy, thus creating and delivering a good life within you. You need to admit that there are problems that you cannot change. But you can change the way of your thinking if you identify the main reason of the problem. And if you acknowledge the facts, that you have been negative or inactive in finding a solution to the problem, probably this will make it easier for you to become positive thus creating a new lease of life within you. You must try to make goals. Making goals can give you a more positive outlook on life. People often tend to get bored with life and get the feeling that they are stuck to negative things which the result they often get the feeling of being depressed. Setting a direction for yourself and a goal would surely help you to move forward. If you expecting to succeed, and are not afraid of failure, you have the best chance of staying positive and can create a very positive life within you. When you, or any of your associates, are tempted to worry about a problem, write out the solution and a definite answer to it. This helps a positive feeling to generate within you. Another thing you need to understand is that there are several ways to cultivate a mental attitude that can bring you peace and happiness and can carnage a good life within you. More of it if you fill your mind with thoughts of peace, courage, health, and hope, your life will be easy to live. You would get a happy feeling of life and mind.

If you let yourself to forget your own unhappiness, by
trying to create a little happiness for others. You are best to
yourself. The perfect way to conquer worry is the Prayer of
God. To keep yourself from worrying about criticism, do
not even try to get mixed with your enemies, because if you
do you will hurt yourself far more than we hurting them.
Instead of worrying about ingratitude, let's expect it. Let's
remember that the only way to find happiness is not to
expect gratitude, but to give for the joy of giving. Let us
build a happy life within us generate peace and a healthy
atmosphere around us. This will help us to lead a peaceful
happy and prosperous life and we would find ourselves to
be happier than before. You should do things in the order of
their importance. You need to clear your desk of all papers
except those relating to the immediate problem at hand.
When you face a problem, solve it then and there, if you
have the facts to make a decision. Make a decision fast and
do not linger on. Learn to organize, deputize, and supervise
and straight away come to decision. Simply postponing it
would spoil your good thoughts and there is every
likelihood your mind may get into negative activities and
start thinking in negative manner. Therefore write down a
list of things that make you excited, however big, small,
likely or unlikely. Then work to make them occur more
often. Look for moments of joy and savor them. Recognize
your good happening every day. Eat well do plenty of
exercise and do not skip meals It is a known fact that
Physical exercise is known to stimulate our veins and get to
strengthen our minds that lift depression and anxiety so we
need to walk, swim, run or whatever we like doing best.

Those who create or those who do well on the worst
scenario, give themselves worry and stress, tend to be
devastated. If we cannot get some sunshine, we can always
lighten up our rooms with brighter lights. We can have
lunch outside the office. Take frequent walks instead of
driving our cars over short distances. No man is
indispensable. First of all our circle of friends is always
there to give us some moral support. Spending time and
engaging ourselves in worthwhile activities could give us a
very enjoyable and satisfying feeling. Nothing feels better
than having group support. Good friends are quite
important and their company generally lightened up our
spirits. To get to know and to find such friends we simply
have to be friendly with ourselves, and then the friendships
will naturally follow us. We need to understand the power
of touch and support and we have not to underestimate it
strength and support. Don't we feel so good when someone
pats us on our back and gives us some words of
encouragement during your most challenging times and
difficult times? Just hug or embrace someone someday you
will see that you have almost changed his life. Get intimate
with him and try to establish close ties with his family and
friends. The love and care expressed by you will
tremendously boost him and well as your immune system
and fury of worry will be diminished for all. In our lives
storms may come and go in the form of reversals, but if we
have the power and foundation of inner fulfillment and if
we deal with it with a very clear practical mind these
storms will not kill us or will not disrupt us. There could be
numberless reasons for which we keep on worrying. We
may be worried about our health, wealth, loved ones,

friends, the happening f yesterday and the follow happenings of tomorrow, the environment or the world politics, but these can be dealt with firm mind and fearless worry if we generate within ourselves the power of enlightenment within ourselves.

LEAVE WORRIES NOW
BE HAPPY ENJOY LIFE

CHAPTER 30

ANALYZING GOOD AND HAPPY LIVING

Annalise sweet good and happy living and stop worrying over petty matters. Generate sweet living and generate good thoughts. Don't wait around or expect others to create happiness that is entirely yours to make. Whatever your goal is, do whatever you have to do to get it, always keep yourself to be a happy person. Why worry about the future. Just imagine as to what if we just acted like everything was easy and there was nothing very serious about it to come in future. Worry often gives a small thing a big shadow and its surrounding do frightened with more scary things with the result we do not tend to have a happy life or a sweet and happing living.

Make yourself aware of what's possible in this world.

Worrying will carry tomorrow's load with today's strength. Worry will not empty tomorrow of its sorrows, but it tends to empty today of its power and strength. Worries make you to move into tomorrow ahead of time. Half the worry in the world is caused by people trying to make decisions before they have sufficient knowledge on which to base a decision. Their negative thoughts pressurise them to be away from the positivity in their lives as they fail and do not analysis on positive and they fail to lead a happy life or sweet life.

Why worry about tomorrow;

Concentrate on today happening as for tomorrow will worry about itself. Each day has its own worries and troubles. Always think that you are a happy man. If there is not any solution to the some problem then do not waste time worrying about it. And if there is a solution to the problem then why waste time worrying about it. Act fast be happy generate positive happiness worries will automatically vanish in the air and you are sure to lead a sweet life and happy life.

The first step to good and happy is by way of creating good and happy thoughts in your minds.

Focus your imagination and make efforts on becoming new positive person. Create happiness in you. Divert your mind to good thoughts. It is much easier to bring about change if you just put your mind to it and change your thoughts into a much more positive direction. We know that it is difficult for us to control things that happen in our lives, but we can, with some effort, control what we think or do in our lives. Positive thoughts will make our imagination livelier and we would be able to lead our lives happily without many worries.

The second good step is to have the company of good and positive living friends.

Appreciate the people in your life who have stood by you through thick and thin. Count their support and analyses the happiness in them which will help you to lead a much happier life.

Good friends help each other in the days of crises and through both the good and bad times. Keep yourself busy and surround yourself with good friends, who always think positive. Feel positive about them and feel lucky to have them in your company. Share positive thoughts with them. Tell them to be happy and to lead a sweet good and happy life.

The third step is to focus your imagination on happy things in life by giving a good smile.

The easiest way is feeling happy. Many theories have revealed that happiness can lift one's mood and can divert your mind to sweet living. We may also share positivity with others by flashing them with a brilliant and good smile. Positive and sweet talks are the rewards of good and happy thoughts it generates more happiness. Dejection, disappointments and depression, however, have consequences that could ruin our health, and life. We must divert their minds to focus to the imagination of good and happy life. If something bad or good is to happen it is sure to happen, whether we are sad or unhappy or depressed. Let us put our energy into today and stop worrying about the future and past. We should not foresee trouble, or worry about what may never happen as past is dead and gone forever and future is uncertain and yet to come. Be your unabashed self in all the best ways that you can.

The basic facts we should know about happiness.

The basic techniques to analyze happiness and how to break the unhappy habits before it breaks us.

These are the simple ways where we can concentrate and get rid of unhappy thoughts. Annalise unhappiness to see and get the reasons and facts as to why we worry. To avoid reoccurrence of worries, concentrate on prayers as prayers are the best source of remedies of the prevailing worries. The more you pray, the less you'll panic. The more you worship, the less you worry. There is nothing that wastes the body like worry, and anyone who has any faith in God should need not to worry about anything whatsoever is to happen in future. This will ease our way to a sweet good and happy living.

What do we think about happy thoughts?

The feeling of happiness   is within us. It is said that sweet good and happy living is purely our own matter and it has nothing to do with our external circumstances. There is something very special within us which keeps us happy and there is something very unpleasant within us which keeps unhappy. Yes quite true it is the positiveness within us that make and creates happiness within us Happy living through positivity is nothing more than that of living a normal life free from undue pressures, problems and tensions. If we want to live a happy life then we need to get rid of the negativity and we must try to avoid all the unpleasant things within us which makes us unhappy.

Negative approach always complicates the problems and increases unhappiness.

Most of us do the fatal mistake of looking outwards for happiness rather than looking inwards. Be happy, be strong, be bold and be courageous every day.

Even if we are having a bad day, think of some good things that may come our way, either later that day, tomorrow, next week, month, or next moment. When everything seems to be beyond our control, it's almost too easy for us to slip into the grasp of unhappiness. To avoid unhappiness we must strive to abolish this sort of thinking through the power of thinking positively. We ought to know the basic fundamental of analyzing happiness. Worries and unhappiness create unnecessary thoughts and these are caused by people going in for unwanted decisions, fore hand not even knowing as to when a good decision is made and not even having sufficient knowledge about it.

Simply making castles in the air won't solve our problems.

We must first study and after carefully weighing all the facts than only come to a powerful decision. Simply making castles in the air won't solve our problems but add more to our vows and unhappiness which may even lead us to unhappy life. Anxiety and worry can go hand in hand. When anxiety grabs the mind, it is self-perpetuating. Your mind gets clogged with numerous buts and ifs. Do not worry about your life.

LEAVE WORRIES NOW
BE HAPPY ENJOY LIFE

CHAPTER 31

WORRIES ARE REPETITIVE THOUGHTS

Negativity and worries are repetitive thoughts associated with feelings of anxiety in anticipation of some negative future event. Worries and anxious feelings lead to disasters and make our lives unhappy. If we know that our circumstances are beyond our control or power we need to change them or revise them to our liking. We must try to put a stop-less order on our worries. We must be careful and we need not permit little things which become insects of our lives to ruin our happiness. Co-operate with the inevitable. Decide just how much anxiety a thing may be worth and refuse to give in anymore. All the happiness is not given in one go it comes slowly and slowly. We must pay special attention to remain happy and be happy. Keep ourselves happy, treat our worried thoughts as valuable signals to a sweet living good and happy living.

The utmost cause of unhappiness is your state of depression. Unhappiness is not there to motivate information gathering or problem-solving. In fact it is depression that constructs the future of unhappiness. Depression is inertia. That's the thing about depression: depression is so insidious, and it compounds daily, and it's impossible to ever see the end of it.

Keep yourself happy

Depressed people think they know themselves, but maybe they only know depression. There are no hopeless than this to get depressed create unhappiness in our minds and become unhappy all the time. Our attitude towards suffering and depression becomes very important because it can affect how we cope with suffering when it arises. Depression is nourished by a lifetime of grieved and unforgiven causes. Another factor to remain unhappy is worrying about unwanted and useless things. Worry is a misuse of the imagination. To keep yourself happy, treat your worried thoughts as most unwanted assets. These are the fundamental facts you should be familiar about worries. A huge factor to stay happy is to cater your worries around, an important relationship in your life and pay special attention sustaining positive relationships. Make your mind firm and do come to a positive decision and not allow the worries to un-ease the power your mind and soul that can cause unhappiness in you.

We must free ourselves from fruitless worry.

Once a decision is carefully reached we should get busy carrying out our decisions and should not bother about all the anxieties that are about to come. When we, or any of our colleagues or associates, are about to worry about a problem, we must write it out and think of the following questions: Instead of worrying about what people say, why not spend time trying to accomplish something they may admire. What if we just acted like everything was easy? How would your life be different if we stopped worrying about things we can't control and started focusing on the things we can? Let today be the day.

We must free ourselves from fruitless worry, seize the day and take effective action on things we can change thus we would see that our lives changes for the betterment and we are on the right path of a sweet, good and happy living.

STEPS FOR HAPPY LIFE AND POSITIVE LIFE

The secret of successful and happy life lies in keeping ourselves smiling and the character which is the foremost important reason that lies within us. Do not be curious about anything, but in everything, by prayer and petition, with thanksgiving, present your requests to God. Whenever your mind is tempted to jump the fence and start to worry, say this verse aloud or to yourself. You may even have to repeat it over and over again. Am I constantly striving to see the positive in every aspect of my life?. Steps for a successful and happy life. At time we may think that there is no road is left for us from where we can achieve the happiness of our lives. We may also feel that life has become terrible for us to live and we are carrying new hope that someone would come to rescue us. There may be chances that someone who was there with us before might have held on to us when we were on the dark side of the life. We should not forget that happiness in life comes through the doors of positive thoughts; we need to have them first. If one door happen to close, another opens, in the event only when we are confident and optimistic. We have so many reasons to cry and at the same time plenty of reasons to smile as well. Similarly, happiness does not stand for anything, but is on our way of thinking that how do we keep ourselves happy in life. Failure and disappointment are part of our life. The only thing is that we need to face and solve the problem is by keeping our dreams and hope alive be it a reason that success and happiness will come our way again.

The experience has taught us that we should buy some strength, hope and positivity from our loved ones to help ourselves in such a situation rather than surrendering as life is a precious gift of God. What if when everything goes wrong and all the doors of happiness are closed our live becomes a silent. It is a quite common and we are aware of a marvelous proverb that Life itself is a stage and we all are the performers, performing different acts assigned to us by our almighty power. We should not forget as to what is in our possession if it is to fulfill our duties towards our responsibility and do whatever is correct and is allowed by us in our life? However, despite of all these good thoughts which are embodied to us by the almighty fail to revive these unwanted circumstances that lead us to sorrow and difficulties and a situation where we do not know what is correct and good for us and what is wrong for us. We should always remember that, "Life is there, where there is hope". That single thing that remains in our hands is to find out ways to know how to overcome these worries of our life at that very moment when all doors are closed for us which means that whatever situation is there, we must not give up hope. We must fight because there have been always a chance that with good faith and hard work we can turn the odds in our favor. It is often said that it is very easy to advice but when it comes to us, things go out of our control and we fail to suggest a way out for ourselves. We fall into the trap of unnecessary worries and elope ourselves with negative thoughts. We feel better when somebody else is facing some difficulty but when it comes to us we fail to gather that faith, will power and the words of strength. It is a common fact that no one in this world is free of obstacles or difficulties. If all the openings of happiness are shut for us and we have to overcome that and have no way to come out, but to survive lest we must have to learn to swim out of the sorrows because this is what is called life and sorrow free living.

There are lot more examples and in many other situations, where we will find that how we could have faced and fought with our sorrows and difficulties of life when there was no hope left in our lives. When the power of will is at the worst and each one of us knows that the one who is gone never comes back. Neither a thousands of words would not be enough to bring him back nor a million tears, because each and every moment, eyes would only shed tears , mind would remain tensed and we would be simply surrounded by worries and the life seems to have been vanished. Life is ever expanding, contraction is death. As commonly said by big saints that the self- seeking man who is looking after his personal comforts and leading a lazy life for himself there would be no room for him even in the hell and he simply have lost the power of his will. We are quite aware of the fact that faith in oneself is the history of a man and that faith calls the quality of superiority within a person. One cannot do anything without it. We fail only when we do not try very hard to achieve the power and faith within us. As soon as we lose faith, death comes in our way and we are surrounds by all the evils and stupid worries of the world. The secret and history of every successful man is to have, good confidence, faith and strength behind him and that remain the right cause of his single success in life. Unselfishness plays a very vital role in his life. He may not have been perfectly unselfish, yet he was tending towards it. If he had been perfectly unselfish, he would have been as great a success. The degree of unselfishness marks the degree of success everywhere and he leads to be successful man without fear worries and selfishness. There are quite a number of reasons to believe that for a successful and happy life the mystery surrounding it lies in our interests, and good memory which is the basis of our interest, power of desire and aim, keeping ourselves smiling and the doubt free character which is the foremost important reason for a successful and happy life.

If we possess one solid unselfish and doubt free character within ourselves we would be quite happy and successful. The love for God and worshipping God adds to one common thing the immense faith in Him. There may be different beliefs and ways to worship God in different communities, places and religions, but one thing remains the same and that is the Love of God for all of us. Our world is full of odds and evens, happiness and sorrows, fulfilment and emptiness. And these are all created by the Almighty. However, the most beautiful Gift of God, is Human, which is such a mystery driven by Him which could hardly be defined or explained in depth. We know that life cannot be foreseen. Life is not a bed of roses. Life is a battle field and not a bed of roses as every man on earth has to struggle very hard in making his life happy. If aim of our life is to stay happy and let others to be happy, we will be happy and remembered by all. But no one will actually remember us for the wealth we have gained, or success we have achieved. I have no aim in life. Summary living with no purpose in life is just like a feather moving towards the wind. Both career and purpose are different issues but it is equally important to understand the value of these things which would ultimately add spicy flavor to your living .Innovation at work place is what it necessary is how well we judge our work, how good we like and enjoy it. If we take our work as a stiff challenge and as learning everyday then we would start loving it and giving our best. However, if we just work for the sake of then nothing is realized and we do not remain happy in life. Life is such a special gift of Almighty and it is not gifted by Him to use it the way we like or love to. The actual path shown by Him needs to be followed by us for us to reach the peak of betterment every moment. We need to have some positive attitude to look at it comfortably but at the same time having a positive mental attitude does not mean banishing all negative thoughts and people from your life.

The same is true with thoughts. When we go to field with negative thoughts, we banish one and another one arises. Therefore creation of positivity in life is utmost necessary to enjoy the special gift of God to us. Now let's us imagine that we are not feeling at our best today, and we are having thoughts that could be classified as negative. We shouldn't be thinking such negative thoughts. We don't like the negative thoughts. We ought to know that negative thoughts are stressful, demoralizing and depressing. We shouldn't aim to have negative thoughts at all. Often we feel uncomfortable because we think we have to say or do something in response to another person's words. When we find ourselves thinking this way, it helps enormously to take a few moments to check inside and notice what we are feeling. We are deeply depressed that negativity has governed us and has taken a deep root in our minds. If we want to live a positive, joyful life, we must not be surrounded by negative people who don't encourage our happiness. As a negative person, we ought to get attracted too negative people only. Only when we decide to make the change to live a more positive life, we have to get rid of our lives of the most negative influences in it. We are quite aware of the fact that no one is perfect and perfection isn't the goal when it comes to positivity but there were people in our lives who were consistently negative, who constantly bring us down, we need to stop spending so much time with them. We can very well imagine, it is not easy for us to get away from these negative people. It can hurt us to keep distance from people even when you know they aren't good for us and for our current lifestyle. In addition to removing negative influences from them, we also have to get rid of some of our own negative behaviors, such as the drug and alcohol abuse. We need to take some concrete steps and examine which behaviors are good for us and which were not harmful.

What we need is to learn to focus on the positive things, such as working on positive activities and cultivating new, positive relationships. We must let go of the negative ones. This process may be not easy to live a positive life when negative people and behaviors continually pull us down. In every situation or in every person there is something good. Most of the time it's not easy to find the positive qualities but we have to look hard to discover positivity in them. Now, when we are faced with a difficult or challenging situation, we need to think and talk to ourselves and console our mind, no matter how terrible the situation might seem, we can always find something good if we take the time to think about it. It is quite obvious that anything good and bad is learning experience so, at the very least, we must learn from bad experiences. However, there's usually even more to it than that. If you really take some time to have a look at it, we would find something good, something genuinely positive, about every person or situation. Once we start thinking more positively, we will realize that we had to reinforce these thoughts and behaviors within ourselves so that we could stick to it. As with any sort of training, the more we practice, the better we get to be positive. The best and easiest way to do this is to be positive when it comes to who we are. We need to speak to ourselves that we are awesome. And we have done a good job at work thus creating positivity within us. We need to be honest with ourselves, and we need to do our best to look for the good. And, whatever we do, we must not focus on the negative. It is alright not to like everything about ourselves, but don't focus on what we don't like. We have all the positive attributes, and it's up to us to remind ourselves of them every day. Not only do we need to be positive with ourselves for this multiple action to take effect, but we need to be more positive with others. We have to share our wealth of positivity with the people of the world.

The best way is to be nice with other people, no matter what. Tell them that they look nice today. Appreciate their job and tell them that have done a great job on that assignment. Be positive and tell your elder or your kids how much you love them and how great they are. When someone is feeling down, do what we need to do is to cheer him or her up. Do send them gifts nice flower and glow them with nice notes.

LEAVE WORRIES NOW
BE HAPPY ENJOY LIFE

CHAPTER 32

WE MUST LEARN TO SWIM OUT OF SORROWS

It is a common fact that no one in this world is free of obstacles or difficulties. If all the openings of happiness are shut for us and we have to overcome that and have no way to come out, but to survive lest we must have to learn to swim out of the sorrows because this is what is called life and sorrow free living. There are lot more examples and in many other situations, where we will find that how we could have faced and fought with our sorrows and difficulties of life when there was no hope left in our lives.

Fighting for survival is what is needed at odd intervals.

Once we start thinking more positively and happily, we will realize that we had to reinforce these thoughts and behaviors within ourselves so that we could stick to it. As with any sort of training, the more we practice, the better we get to be positive. The best and easiest way to do this is to be positive when it comes to who we are. We need to speak to ourselves that we are awesome. And we have done a good job at work thus creating positivity within us. We need to be honest with ourselves, and we need to do our best to look for the good. And, whatever we do, we must not focus on the negative but focus as to how we can become happy by discarding all negative thoughts and have the feeling to remain happy and gay.

It is alright not to like everything about ourselves, but don't focus on what we don't like. We have all the positive attributes, and it's up to us to remind ourselves of them every day in order to make us to live happily in our lives.

Life is such a special gift of Almighty so always be happy

Life is such a special gift of Almighty and it is not gifted by Him to use it the way we like or love to. The actual path shown by Him needs to be followed by us for us to reach the peak of betterment every moment. We need to have some happy attitude to look at it comfortably but at the same time having a positive mental attitude does not mean banishing all negative thoughts and people from your life. The same is true with thoughts. When we go to field with negative thoughts, we banish one and another one arises. Therefore creation of positivity and creation of happiness in life is utmost necessary to enjoy the special gift of God to us.

Do not create unnecessary worries.

If we try to change the way we look, talk and behave just to please others, and show our pride we will gradually become such a person that we ourselves won't recognize each other and would start and create unnecessary worries within us and our surrounding without being positive and will not start to live happily. Thus we must behave in such a manner so as not to create unnecessary worries in our thoughts and mind. We ought to stop worrying over unnecessary things be positive and live without fear happily.

We need to understand that what people think of us is their concern, and not ours. If they think about us to be, too reticent or proud, it's really not our business. If every time we happen to meet some new fellows, we may wonder and imagine as what they think of us, and with this feeling in us we will never be able to live a trouble-free and hassle free life. We are bound to fall into the trap of unnecessary worries denying us the startup of new and the happy living life. We would not be able to lead a sweet good and happy life. The main reason is that we must think rationally. Is it in our hands or can we control what others think about us? Simply we need to ignore them. If we cannot, and live our lives the way we want to and find the ways to leave worries aside and start living a happy life. Let us make our way to happy living.

Happy Living with Positive Attitudes.

Positive thinking is not about putting on a pair of rose-colored glasses and ignoring all the negative things you will encounter in life. That approach can be just as devastating as ignoring the positive and only focusing on the negative.

Balance, with a healthy dose of realism, is the key. It is a well-known fact that attitude decides how a natives or persons copes up with the day to day events of life. Attitude is what a influence a person's reaction to a situation in life is. It sets the emotional undertone for a person to his likes or dislikes a situation even before he is acquainted with it. Positive attitude is a quality that is second to none in a human being.

Though we attach so much importance to this attitude, as we grow into teenage and adult years we find ourselves becoming ungrateful or taking things for granted. We lose touch with the very same qualities that we instill in our children. We take for granted our life, our health, our families, the people in our lives, the things that our loved ones do for us to make our lives easier and things that we possess.

The positive attitude and happy face speaks a lot about a person.

It denotes about changing negative happiness and making positive thinking and living a positive attitude a good habit. Thinking positively and a positive attitude help us to appreciate and value ourselves, our potential and all that we have. It ensures that we do not take our abilities for granted. It makes us look at ourselves as special people with a special set of abilities and potential. It banishes the feelings of inadequacy and insecurity that arises from unfair comparisons with others. It helps us to appreciate people for who they are and not magnify what they are not and their little flaws. It drives away prejudice and makes us approach life with an open mind. It predisposes us to react to the daily events of life in a positive manner and help us to look at the brighter side of life. Make us optimistic. It gives hope and helps us look forward to life with anticipation and makes us to live happily. We need to know that positive thinking takes the focus away from what we don't have, to appreciating and making good use of what we have. It is closely connected to our emotional wellbeing and happiness.

We feel loved and at peace with ourselves for a major part of our lives when we make this attitude ours. This adds and helps us to get rid of greed, amenity, bitterness, jealousy, and promotes a healthy and nurturing attitude towards others, which in turn gets reciprocated and we feel the sense of healthy living. We attach so much importance to this attitude of gratitude that when our children fail to thank someone, we insist that they do it. That is what is needed to be avoided from time to time. We expect this in return from others when we help them or give them a gift. We call a person discourteous and rude when they do not say thank us in return. On the face of it we ought to know that a positive is not an attitude of being satisfied and content, that you never want to do anything, anymore. This is an attitude that makes you feel good about who you are, what you do, and what your potentials are. This attitude impels you to utilize all that you are endowed with as a person, to achieve the highest possible goals. When we have this attitude, we are able to work without any external pressure to perform but there is sufficient pressure and motivation from within.

The possessing of happy living is like any other habit.

The possessing of happy living is like any other habit, so you need to follow the routine of habit formation here as well. You will win new friends and admirers without having to impress them or conform to the pressure of doing things their way. You will be bubbling with life. You will be rearing to go and accomplish all you can with your new found confidence.

The best part of adopting the 'happy living" is a positive attitude of gratitude is that, you will be able to enjoy the smallest pleasures of nature with a heightened sense of satisfaction and awe. You can see and watch a beautiful flower and carry that joy in your mind for future enjoyment with a clear positive habit. You can go back to work freshen and can use it as an object to meditate on when you feel stressed. You can converge to form of happy living with this habit of positive and sweet living. You need to remember that the possession of happy living is like any other habit and one need not practice so hard to get it. Let us be clear that a positive is not an attitude of being satisfied and content, that we never want to do anything, anymore. This is an attitude that makes you feel good about who you are, what you do, and what your potentials are. This attitude impels you to utilize all that you are endowed with as a person, to achieve the highest possible goals. When we have this attitude, we are able to work without any external pressure to perform but there is sufficient pressure and motivation from within. The habit of happy living is like any other habit, so we need to follow the routine of habit formation here as well.

Keeping our dreams and hope alive our success and happiness.

We should not forget that happiness in life comes through the doors of positive thoughts; we need to have them first. If one door happen to close, another opens, in the event only when we are confident and optimistic. We have so many reasons to cry and at the same time plenty of reasons to smile as well.

Similarly, happiness does not stand for anything, but is on our way of thinking that how do we keep ourselves happy in life. Failure and disappointment are part of our life. The only thing is that we need to face and solve the problem is by keeping our dreams and hope alive be it a reason that success and happiness will come our way again. The experience has taught us that we should buy some strength, hope and positivity from our loved ones to help ourselves in such a situation rather than surrendering as life is a precious gift of God and is equipped with full of joy and happiness if we help ourselves in these critical moments we can live with considerable optimism.

Life is there, where there is hope.

What if when everything goes wrong and all the doors of happiness are closed our live becomes a silent. It is a quite common and we are aware of a marvelous proverb that, Life itself is a stage and we all are the performers, performing different acts assigned to us by our almighty power. We should always remember that, "Life is there, where there is hope". That single thing that remains in our hands is to find out ways to know how to overcome these worries of our life at that very moment when all doors are closed for us which means that whatever situation is there, we must not give up hope. We must fight because there have been always a chance that with good faith and hard work we can turn the odds in our favor. It is often said that it is very easy to advice but when it comes to us, things go out of our control and we fail to suggest a way out for ourselves. We fall into the trap of unnecessary worries and elope ourselves with negative thoughts.

We feel better when somebody else is facing some
difficulty but when it comes to us we fail to gather that
faith, will power and the words of strength. When the
power of will is at the worst and each one of us knows that
the one who is gone never comes back. Neither a thousands
of words would not be enough to bring him back nor a
million tears, because each and every moment, eyes would
only shed tears , mind would remain tensed and we would
be simply surrounded by worries and the life seems to have
been vanished. Life is ever expanding, contraction is death.
As commonly said by big saints that the self- seeking man
who is looking after his personal comforts and leading a
lazy life for himself there would be no room for him even
in the hell and he simply have lost the power of his will.
We are quite aware of the fact that faith in oneself is the
history of a man and that faith calls the quality of
superiority within a person. One cannot do anything
without it. We fail only when we do not try very hard to
achieve the power and faith within us. As soon as we lose
faith, death comes in our way and we are surrounds by all
the evils and stupid worries of the world. The secret and
history of every successful man is to have, good
confidence, faith and strength behind him and that remain
the right cause of his single success in life. Unselfishness
plays a very vital role in his life. He may not have been
perfectly unselfish, yet he was tending towards it. If he had
been perfectly unselfish, he would have been as great a
success. The degree of unselfishness marks the degree of
success everywhere and he leads to be successful man
without fear worries and selfishness.

There are quite a number of reasons to believe that for a successful and happy life the mystery surrounding it lies in our interests, and good memory which is the basis of our interest, power of desire and aim, keeping ourselves smiling and the doubt free character which is the foremost important reason for a successful and happy life. If we possess one solid unselfish and doubt free character within ourselves we would be quite happy and successful.

The love for God and worshipping.

The love for God and worshipping God adds to one common thing the immense faith in Him. There may be different beliefs and ways to worship God in different communities, places and religions, but one thing remains the same and that is the Love of God for all of us. Our world is full of odds and evens, happiness and sorrows, fulfilment and emptiness. And these are all created by the Almighty. However, the most beautiful Gift of God, is a Human, which is such a mystery driven by Him which could hardly be defined or explained in depth.

The secret of successful and happy life lies in keeping ourselves smiling.

The secret of successful and happy life lies in keeping ourselves smiling and the character which is the foremost important reason that lies within us. Do not be curious about anything, but in everything, by prayer and petition, with thanksgiving, present your requests to God. Whenever your mind is tempted to jump the fence and start to worry, say this verse aloud or to yourself. You may even have to repeat it over and over again.

Steps for a successful and happy life.

Being a positive thinker is not about ignoring reality in favor of aspirational thoughts. It is more about taking a proactive approach to your life. Instead of feeling hopeless or overwhelmed, positive thinking allows you to tackle life's challenges by looking for effective ways to resolve conflict and come up with creative solutions to problems.

LEAVE WORRIES NOW
BE HAPPY ENJOY LIFE

CHAPTER 33

LIFE IS NOT BED OF ROSES

Life is a battle field and not a bed of roses as every man on earth has to struggle very hard in making his life happy. If aim of our life is to stay happy and let others to be happy, we will be happy and remembered by all. But no one will actually remember us for the wealth we have gained, or success we have achieved. If we have no aim in life, we would not be able to lead and happy life. Living with no purpose in life is just like a feather moving towards the wind. Both career and purpose are different issues but it is equally important to understand the value of these things which would ultimately add spicy flavor to your living. Innovation at work place is what is it necessary how well we judge our work, how good we like and enjoy it. If we take our work as a stiff challenge and as learning everyday then we would start loving it and giving our best. However, if we just work for the sake of then nothing is realized and we do not remain happy in life.

We should not aim to have negative thoughts at all.

Now let's us imagine that we are not feeling at our best today, and we are having thoughts that could be classified as negative. We shouldn't be thinking such negative thoughts. We don't like the negative thoughts.

We ought to know that negative thoughts are stressful,
demoralizing and depressing. We shouldn't aim to have
negative thoughts at all. Often we feel uncomfortable
because we think we have to say or do something in
response to another person's words. When we find
ourselves thinking this way, it helps enormously to take a
few moments to check inside and notice what we are
feeling. Negative thoughts destroy our happy livings. We
ought to discard all these negative thought and act to live in
a more positive atmosphere rather than living in a negative
world where we can never find a happy living.

Positivity is state of mind

Positivity is something you cannot earn or buy. If you have
spent your life trying to get some happiness or something
that will make you happy, odds are that you are wasting a
really good life that you don't know you have. You passed
up and overlooked a lot of personal happiness. You are
probably spending so much time chasing and dreaming of
unnecessary thing of what could be of no use to you and
that you are forgetting about all the small and big things
occurring right now that could make you happy. People and
things alone, won't make you happy. Your own efforts not
to get worried or depressed make you happy. You know the
saying, that "Positivity is a state of mind". And state of
mind is what you think do and act in a peaceful manner
without being getting worried or depressed. The best thing
about happiness is that you get it is free. You don't have to
pay or you do not have to open any account to be happy.
You don't have to pay monthly rent for it either. You just
have to change your perspective, your views on what you
are seeing and feeling.

Happiness is not something which is quite readymade. It comes from your own actions and deeds. Don't let one cloud darken the whole sky. Angriness and happiness don't mix. You must dig out the angriness in you, and see that the happiness has shown and seeded a place to grow its roots. The ultimate goal of life should be to get happiness and not get involved into unnecessary worries falling in the death trap of defeats and failures. The essence of life is not in the great victories and grand failures, but in the simple joys. The purpose of our lives is to be happy. Laugh when you can, apologize when you should, and let go of what you can't change. Think positive and just visualize that what is stored in destiny would not be negative. If you want to be happy, be positive first practice meditation. If you want, others to be happy practice compassion. Whoever is happy will make others happy, too. Let us be very sure and let us keep in mind that happiness doesn't depend on any superficial conditions, it is governed by our mental attitude only. Our greatest gift to others is to be happy and to radiate our happiness to the entire world. Happiness is a guide to direction, not a place to hide. As a happy person, you radiate happiness to the world. Visualize your light radiating throughout the world, passing from person to person until it encircles the globe. Resolve to keep happy, and your joy and you shall form an invincible host against difficulties. The positive persons often dance to the happy tunes of their lives. The path to happiness is forgiveness of everyone and gratitude for everything. Happiness fills your heart each day and your whole life through with clean thoughts. Any day would be a wonderful day if you do not to take life so seriously.

Happiness is not about being a winner -it's about being gentle with life being gentle within you. Happiness blooms in the presence of self-respect and the absence of ego. Love yourself. Love everyone around you. Love everyone in the whole world. When you're feeling depressed or anxious, close your eyes and try to visualize a guided positive imaginary thing. First breathe deeply and relax. How important it is to consistently reach for positive, uplifting, inspirational thoughts. Thought that promote aliveness and abundance. Thoughts that make you feel good. Look at the birds of the air; they do not sow or reap or store away in barns, and yet our heavenly Father feeds them. Imagine that you're already a positive person and you love life. The only thing between us and our desire, to be happy, is one single fact: we are not happy because we often fall into the death trap of depression and wholly because of our negative thoughts. Absence of positive thinking, has eluded us of our great happiness and left us far behind. This very little known fact has kept many of us from reaching our goal of happiness. If you keep thinking things like as if your life is dead!", nothing would be achieved and it will be like that only. Throw away all your negative thoughts and worries, concentrate on the goals to be achieved, on the ray of happiness in you and make sure that you are not falling again into the path of negativity. "Happiness is a state of mind only and not the thoughts of negatives, and it quite true that happiness can only be achieved if you have a positive mind and a clear attitude of being a positive person. Happiness and positivity go hand in hand.

If you are positive you are a happy person and if you possess negativity you would land yourself to be a very negative person thus ruining your life for what of nothing.

Have Positive Thinking

Have Positive Thinking, think positive as all your thoughts, good and bad, are the creation of your mind which tends to lead you to a materialistic life and go in to generate unnecessary worries. Thus you will learn to be more positive. The environment and all the experiences in your life are the results of your habitual and dominant thoughts. Positive thoughts bring good and happiness. Negative thoughts could tell us about something that needs special attention when they lead us to the path of worries. We must discover what needs to be done, and think positively to take care of it. Many of us fail to see a negative occurrence and do not think of a replacement of negative thought with positive one. As they even do not even dare look for a bright side in every situation. If we do this for a longer period of time, we become habitual, and it will make a tremendous delay in improving our positive thinking skills. We must remember, everything can be framed positively if we make a restless effort to do so. Positive thinking wards off the ingredients of negative thoughts in our minds there are both positive and negative aspects to most situations. We get to choose which ones we will focus on. We can try to catch ourselves when we're being negative and do not try thinking the positive side of the things. There's no sense in worrying about the negatives if these negatives cannot be changed.

If we waste energy and happiness on the things we can't change, we'll only make ourselves more frustrated and come to the stage of depression dejection and disappointments. Negativity is a habit and we often don't realize we're doing ourselves down. Under each negative thought that we have written, we can spot an alternative way of looking at it, that isn't so negative. Take your mind to positivity and mold and drive your thoughts to the positivity. There's a world of difference between expecting failure or rejection so as not to be disappointed when it occurs and recognizing it as a possibility of being positive. It's sensible to look at a situation from all angles and to have a back-up plan to fall back on if need be. People who do this will not see failure as another step on the road to eventual success; but by expecting and envisioning success, there's less likely to be a failure. Let us find some ways of removing negative thoughts and discouraging our worries to be born.

The first step is by way of giving a good smile.

The easiest way is smiling. Many theories have revealed that even a forced smile can lift one's mood and can divert your mind to positive thinking.. We may also share positivity with others by flashing them with a brilliant and good smile. Positive Thinking is a reward of good Smiling and not a risk. The only thing we risk when we think positive is giving ourselves a little more happiness.

The second good step is to have the company of positive thinking friends.

Keep yourself busy and surround yourself with good friends, who always think positive. Appreciate the people in your life who have stood by you through thick and thin. Count their support and analyses the positivity in them which will help you to become more positive, and in the process you will probably help them too. Good friends help each other in the days of crises and through both the good and bad times. Feel positive about them and feel lucky to have them in your company. Share positive thoughts with them. Tell them to be more positive in live.

The third step is to focus your imagination on positive thoughts

Focus your imagination and make efforts on becoming new positive person. Create positivizes in you. Divert your mind to positive thinking. It is much easier to bring about change if you just put your mind to it and change your thoughts into a much more positive direction. We know that it is difficult for us to control things that happen in our lives, but we can, with some effort, control what we think or do in our lives. Positive thinking will make our imagination livelier and we would be able to lead our lives without many worries. Dejection, Disappointments and Depression, however, has consequences that could ruin our, health, and well-being. This is the reason why many people suffer from depression much more often in winter than in the other seasons. It's because the days are shorter and do not divert their minds to focus to the imagination of positive thinking.

LEAVE WORRIES NOW
BE HAPPY ENJOY LIFE

CHAPTER 34

CREATE HAPPY LIFE WITHIN YOU.

If you are interested in getting more success and happiness

If you are interested in getting more success and happiness within you, focus on all the ways as if you have already attained success. You need to focus on the thing and create a happy live within you. If you want love and affection, focus on all the people and the abundance of love that you have to give to them. I

f we want to have greater health, focus on all the ways that we are healthy, thus creating and delivering a good life within you. You need to admit that there are problems that you cannot change. But you can change the way of your thinking if you identify the main reason of the problem. And if you acknowledge the facts, that you have been negative or inactive in finding a solution to the problem, probably this will make it easier for you to become positive thus creating a new lease of life within you. It will make your life easier to lead a good and sweet life.

You must try to make goals

You must try to make goals. Making goals can give you a more positive outlook on life.

People often tend to get bored with life and get the feeling that they are stuck to negative things which the result they often get the feeling of being depressed. Setting a direction for yourself and a goal would surely help you to move forward.

Mental attitude that can bring you peace and happiness

If you expecting to succeed, and are not afraid of failure, you have the best chance of staying positive and can create a very positive life within you. When you, or any of your associates, are tempted to worry about a problem, write out the solution and a definite answer to it. This helps a positive feeling to generate within you making you very positive to have a good living. Another thing you need to understand is that there are several ways to cultivate a mental attitude that can bring you peace and happiness and can carnage a good life within you. More of it if you fill your mind with thoughts of peace, courage, health, and hope, your life will be easy to live. You would get a happy feeling of life and mind if you let yourself to forget your own unhappiness, by trying to create a little happiness for others. You are best to yourself and to others.

The first step is to write down your worries

The first step is to write down your worries, which will help you make sense of them, and then decide on one small step you can take towards a solution. But to be very true no man in this world is free of obstacles or difficulties. Don't make worry your habit. Break this habit and stop all the negative and panic thoughts provoking your mind all the time.

If you can't change the past, but you must not ruin the present by worrying about the future. Joy is what happens to us when we allow ourselves to recognize how good things really are. When we feel worried and depressed, we need to consciously form a smile on our faces and act upbeat until the happy feeling becomes genuine reality. Happiness is what is needed most. What makes to lead a happy life is not to get trapped into unnecessary unwanted worries and negative thoughts.

Don't create the feeling of depression and anger.

Feelings of depression and hopelessness and or anger are even tougher to cope with on a consistent basis. When you are worried, you not only hurt yourself, but the limited support systems that are still holding on your mind but making you to get more and more worried and nothing is achieved in terms of success except the re-carnation of worries and worries thus leading you to be unhappy and worried all the time. Your actions breed confidence and courage. If you want to conquer fear, anger and worry do not sit ideal and just think about it. Let our deep worrying become advance thinking and planning. If you look into your own mind and heart, and you find nothing wrong there, what is there to worry about? Practically nothing what is there to fear about and again nothing? So why worry unnecessarily and make your present and future dark. Neglect all those which make your life unhappy.

Why being a negative person?

Why being a negative person and what do you get out of it being a depression dejected and sad man.?

Why not turn your thoughts to be a positive person simply it is a question of tilting your mind towards a positive side of thing. See both the aspects of a situation and ways the pros and cons of both the sides and try to abolish the negativity in you. Be positive strong and you will remain happy for ever. We all have different roles that we play in the lives of people we love and care about. Our actions and how well we play our part has a direct influence on their life, so we better get in there and give our best performance. Tell them with how much you care in the capacity that you're in. At the end of the day, money is just a means to an end. Nothing more. If you're grinding and struggling to make ends meet and buried under piles of debt, that's pretty stressful. Once you have your basic needs met though, more money only makes you happier up to a certain point. Money cannot buy you happiness. You need to generate it yourself. Someone will always be better than you at something, but it does not matter. Be inspired by them, using it to push yourself further, and nothing more. If they can do it, why cannot you?

Are you are interested in getting more happiness?

If you are interested in getting more happiness focus on all the ways as if you have already attained success. You need to focus on the thing and create a live within you. If you want love and affection, focus on all the people and the abundance of love that you have to give to them.

Worrisome thoughts reproduce faster.

Worrisome thoughts reproduce faster so one of the most powerful ways to stop the spiral of worry is simply to disclose the worry to a friend. Practice happy gratitude daily. Take three minutes at the end of your day to chill and write down a small list of the things that can make you smile, laugh, or that you're glad are a part of your life. There's something to be grateful about, especially when you look down at that list and realize that a lot of people have it worse off than you do and could use a few of those things. Simply being an optimist will not solve all your problems, but what's the alternative is to keep your mind and heart cool and always have happy and positive feeling and think that life is to live happily. There isn't much sense in being anything else. If you're constantly filling your head with negative thoughts, odds are they'll lead you straight towards negative actions, self-doubt and increase the general happiness of life isn't a cool place to live at all. Think of each setback as a challenge to see the positive, spin the situation back around, making it better than it was before and start living in a good and sweet manner.

What do we get out of unhappiness?

We may feel largely uncomfortable, when worries attack our thoughts and mind. While we are consuming more worries we are far too busy to do anything else to fix the real problem and would rather find it hard to get into a smart solution. Thus resulting in a fact that you spend your evenings worrying only without even bothering to find some time to know its cause We get nothing out of worrying except only to think and cry and become unhappy.

We do not get anything out of unhappiness. Another thing is that we may feel largely uncomfortable, when worries attack our thoughts and mind which makes worrying about a situation an easier option to get depressed and diffused. While we are consuming more worries we are far too busy to do anything else to fix the real problem and would rather find it hard to get into a smart solution. Thus resulting in a fact that we spend our evenings worrying only without even bothering to find some time to search a sweet happiness within us.

Negative thoughts create unnecessary worries

Negative thought which are provoking our mind, about the uncertainties and the negativities, as to what will happen tomorrow creates unnecessary worries and worries are repetitive thoughts associated with feelings of anxiety in anticipation of some negative future event which may end in a failure. Whether the worries are about financial crisis, family problems, work, health or any topic of concern, the anxious feelings and negative thoughts produced are always distinctly unpleasant thus making us unhappy all the time. We get nothing being a negative and unhappy man. We must not forget that if we tend to worry they will never rob tomorrow of its sorrows, but will only deny today of its meaning happiness and joys. Negative thoughts only produce worries and worrying is actually a form of superstition and creates false images in our mind and that is the main reason and cause which makes and leads us to this point of imagination.

A human being can survive almost anything, as long as he or she sees the end in sight, starts analyzing his positive thoughts and starts analyzing his unhappiness.

We need to fore see the coming trouble first.

We must not forgot that if something bad or good is to happen it is sure to happen, whether we worry or not. Let us put our energy into today and stop worrying about the future and past. We should not foresee trouble, or worry about what may never happen as past is dead and gone forever and future is uncertain and yet to come. Positive thinking our brave attitude and our courage will ward off everything and bring happiness in our lives. The basic facts we should know about worry. The basic techniques to analyze worry and how to break the worry habit before it breaks us. These are the simple ways where we can concentrate and get rid of worries prevailing in our thoughts, remove all the negativity in our live and start living a positive good and happy life.

Think of good and positive ways of Happy Living.

Annalise positive ways of happy living and get to see the reasons and facts of worry. To avoid reoccurrence of worries, concentrate on prayers as prayers are the best source of remedies of the prevailing worries. Think good ways of living and starting praying. The more you pray, the less you'll panic. The more you worship, the less you worry. There is nothing that wastes the body like worry, and anyone who has any faith in God should need not to worry about anything whatsoever is to happen in future.

Positive thinking is the creation of good imagination and good imagination is the creation of sweet and happy living.

Happiness comes with Positive living and sweet thoughts

If you know that the circumstance is beyond your control or power change than revise it to your liking. Just try to put a stop-less order on your worries. Don't permit little things which become insects of life to ruin your happiness. Co-operate with the inevitable. Decide just how much anxiety a thing may be worth and refuse to give in anymore.

All the happiness is not given in one go it comes slowly and slowly with positive thinking.

Have worry under your control. If your worries center around, pay special attention to remain positive and be happy. Keep yourself happy, treat your worried thoughts as valuable signals. How to keep from worrying about criticism? Simply unjust criticism and think positively and do often discard a bad compliment. It often means that you have aroused jealousy and envy. Let's keep a record of the fool things we have done and stop criticizing ourselves.

Cause of unhappiness is Negative way of living life

The utmost cause of worry is our negative thinking as it leads us to the state of depression. Living will change for the better-If You Think Positive. Our negative thinking and attitude towards suffering and depression becomes very important because it can affect how we cope with suffering when it arises. Depression is nourished by a lifetime of un-grieved and unforgiven causes.

Times will change for the better when you change. Worry is a misuse of the imagination. Worry is most often a prideful way of thinking that you have more control over life and its circumstances than you actually do. Positive Thinking leads your way to good and happiness. An art of Good and Happy Living.

Neglect worries keep yourself happy.

Neglect worries keep yourself happy, treat your worried thoughts as valuable signals. These are the fundamental facts you should be familiar about worries. A huge factor to stay happy is to cater your worries around, an important relationship in your life and pay special attention sustaining positive relationships. Worries are there to motivate information gathering and problem-solving. Make your mind firm and do come to a positive decision as come what we will not allow the worries to entire our mind and soul.

What if we just acted like everything was easy?

Once a decision is carefully reached we should get busy carrying out our decisions and should not bother about all the anxieties that are about to come. When we, or any of our colleagues or associates, are about to worry about a problem, we must write it out and think positively of the questions. Instead of worrying about what people say of you, why not spend time trying to accomplish something they will admire. What if we just acted like everything was easy? How would your life be different if you stopped worrying about things we can't control and started focusing on the things we can? Let today be the day.

Free yourself from fruitless worry, seize the day and take effective action on things you can change. We would change ourselves for the betterment if we start thinking in positive terms. Positive thinking is what is required of us and simply worrying about the future things or as to what will happen in the next moment will certainly deprive us of good and happy living that we are about gather or get in the next hour.

Another cause of getting worried or unhappy is the attachment

Attachment brings worry. If you have a problem and you come up with the answer, you stop worrying immediately. Our minds can be dishonest, persuading us that we are worrying about something, when our deepest fear is entirely different. No-one likes to admit that they've chosen to worry. The first step is to write down your worries, which will help you make sense of them, and then decide on one small step you can take towards a solution. But to be very true no man in this world is free of obstacles or difficulties. Don't make worry your habit. Break this habit and stop all the negative and panic thoughts provoking your mind all the time if you want to remain a happy person and lead a happy good and sweet life. Feelings of depression and angry are even tougher to cope with on a consistent basis. When you are worried, you not only hurt yourself, but the limited support systems that are still holding on your mind making you to get more and more worried and nothing is achieved in terms of success except the re-carnation of worries and worries .

Joy is what happens to us when we allow ourselves to recognize how good things really are.

Practically nothing what is there to fear about?

So why worry unnecessarily and make your present and future dark. Why being a negative person and what do you get out of it being a depression dejected and sad man.? Why not turn your thoughts to be a positive person simply it is a question of tilting your mind towards a positive side of thing. See both the aspects of a situation and ways the pros and cons of both the sides and try to abolish the negativity in you. You will surely be a happy man.

Think of the best the best is sure to happen

Think of the best the best is sure to happen and if you think of the worst the worst will come. Better come forward wake up and think positive first. Positive persons always succeed in life whatever be the circumstances and the negative often dig a death trap for themselves. So why be a negative person why you have all the qualities of being a positive man. Surround yourself with friends and people that are better than you in areas that you want to improve in. Learn from them, let them push you out of your comfort zone and it's only a matter of time before you level up as well. Happiness is neither virtue nor pleasure nor this thing nor that but simply growth. We are happy when we are growing.

LEAVE WORRIES NOW
BE HAPPY ENJOY LIFE

CHAPTER 35

ANALYZING GOOD AND HAPPY LIVING

Annalise sweet good and happy living and stop worrying over petty matters. Generate sweet living and generate good thoughts. Don't wait around or expect others to create happiness that is entirely yours to make. Whatever your goal is, do whatever you have to do to get it, always keep yourself to be a happy person. Why worry about the future. Just imagine as to what if we just acted like everything was easy and there was nothing very serious about it to come in future. Worry often gives a small thing a big shadow and its surrounding do frightened with more scary things with the result we do not tend to have a happy life or a sweet and happing living.

Make yourself aware of what's possible in this world.

Worrying will carry tomorrow's load with today's strength. Worry will not empty tomorrow of its sorrows, but it tends to empty today of its power and strength. Worries make you to move into tomorrow ahead of time. Half the worry in the world is caused by people trying to make decisions before they have sufficient knowledge on which to base a decision. Their negative thoughts pressurise them to be away from the positivity in their lives as they fail and do not analysis on positive and they fail to lead a happy life or sweet life.

Why worry about tomorrow;

Concentrate on today happening as for tomorrow will worry about itself. Each day has its own worries and troubles. Always think that you are a happy man. If there is not any solution to the some problem then do not waste time worrying about it. And if there is a solution to the problem then why waste time worrying about it. Act fast be happy generate positive happiness worries will automatically vanish in the air and you are sure to lead a sweet life and happy life.

The first step to good and happy is by way of creating good and happy thoughts in your minds.

Focus your imagination and make efforts on becoming new positive person. Create happiness in you. Divert your mind to good thoughts. It is much easier to bring about change if you just put your mind to it and change your thoughts into a much more positive direction. We know that it is difficult for us to control things that happen in our lives, but we can, with some effort, control what we think or do in our lives. Positive thoughts will make our imagination livelier and we would be able to lead our lives happily without many worries.

The second good step is to have the company of good and positive living friends.

Appreciate the people in your life who have stood by you through thick and thin. Count their support and analyses the happiness in them which will help you to lead a much happier life.

Good friends help each other in the days of crises and through both the good and bad times. Keep yourself busy and surround yourself with good friends, who always think positive. Feel positive about them and feel lucky to have them in your company. Share positive thoughts with them. Tell them to be happy and to lead a sweet good and happy life.

The third step is to focus your imagination on happy things in life by giving a good smile.

The easiest way is feeling happy. Many theories have revealed that happiness can lift one's mood and can divert your mind to sweet living. We may also share positivity with others by flashing them with a brilliant and good smile. Positive and sweet talks are the rewards of good and happy thoughts it generates more happiness. Dejection, disappointments and depression, however, have consequences that could ruin our health, and life. We must divert their minds to focus to the imagination of good and happy life. If something bad or good is to happen it is sure to happen, whether we are sad or unhappy or depressed. Let us put our energy into today and stop worrying about the future and past. We should not foresee trouble, or worry about what may never happen as past is dead and gone forever and future is uncertain and yet to come. Be your unabashed self in all the best ways that you can.

The basic facts we should know about happiness.

The basic techniques to analyze happiness and how to break the unhappy habits before it breaks us.

These are the simple ways where we can concentrate and get rid of unhappy thoughts. Annalise unhappiness to see and get the reasons and facts as to why we worry. To avoid reoccurrence of worries, concentrate on prayers as prayers are the best source of remedies of the prevailing worries. The more you pray, the less you'll panic. The more you worship, the less you worry. There is nothing that wastes the body like worry, and anyone who has any faith in God should need not to worry about anything whatsoever is to happen in future. This will ease our way to a sweet good and happy living.

What do we think about happy thoughts?

The feeling of happiness   is within us. It is said that sweet good and happy living is purely our own matter and it has nothing to do with our external circumstances. There is something very special within us which keeps us happy and there is something very unpleasant within us which keeps unhappy. Yes quite true it is the positiveness within us that make and creates happiness within us Happy living through positivity is nothing more than that of living a normal life free from undue pressures, problems and tensions. If we want to live a happy life then we need to get rid of the negativity and we must try to avoid all the unpleasant things within us which makes us unhappy.

Negative approach always complicates the problems and increases unhappiness.

Most of us do the fatal mistake of looking outwards for happiness rather than looking inwards. Be happy, be strong, be bold and be courageous every day.

Even if we are having a bad day, think of some good things that may come our way, either later that day, tomorrow, next week, month, or next moment.

Simply making castles in the air won't solve our problems.

When everything seems to be beyond our control, it's almost too easy for us to slip into the grasp of unhappiness. To avoid unhappiness we must strive to abolish this sort of thinking through the power of thinking positively. We ought to know the basic fundamental of analyzing happiness. Worries and unhappiness create unnecessary thoughts and these are caused by people going in for unwanted decisions, fore hand not even knowing as to when a good decision is made and not even having sufficient knowledge about it. We must first study and after carefully weighing all the facts than only come to a powerful decision. Simply making castles in the air won't solve our problems but add more to our vows and unhappiness which may even lead us to unhappy life. Anxiety and worry can go hand in hand. When anxiety grabs the mind, it is self-perpetuating. Your mind gets clogged with numerous buts and ifs. Do not worry about your life.

Negativity and worries are repetitive thoughts

Negativity and worries are repetitive thoughts associated with feelings of anxiety in anticipation of some negative future event. Worries and anxious feelings lead to disasters and make our lives unhappy.

If we know that our circumstances are beyond our control or power we need to change them or revise them to our liking. We must try to put a stop-less order on our worries. We must be careful and we need not permit little things which become insects of our lives to ruin our happiness. Co-operate with the inevitable. Decide just how much anxiety a thing may be worth and refuse to give in anymore. All the happiness is not given in one go it comes slowly and slowly. We must pay special attention to remain happy and be happy. Keep ourselves happy, treat our worried thoughts as valuable signals to a sweet living good and happy living.

The utmost cause of unhappiness is your state of depression. Unhappiness is not there to motivate information gathering or problem-solving. In fact it is depression that constructs the future of unhappiness. Depression is inertia. That's the thing about depression: depression is so insidious, and it compounds daily, and it's impossible to ever see the end of it. Depressed people think they know themselves, but maybe they only know depression. There are no hopeless than this to get depressed create unhappiness in our minds and become unhappy all the time. Our attitude towards suffering and depression becomes very important because it can affect how we cope with suffering when it arises.

Keep yourself happy

Depression is nourished by a lifetime of grieved and unforgiven causes. Another factor to remain unhappy is worrying about unwanted and useless things. Worry is a misuse of the imagination.

To keep yourself happy, treat your worried thoughts as most unwanted assets. These are the fundamental facts you should be familiar about worries. A huge factor to stay happy is to cater your worries around, an important relationship in your life and pay special attention sustaining positive relationships. Make your mind firm and do come to a positive decision and not allow the worries to un-ease the power your mind and soul that can cause unhappiness in you.

We must free ourselves from fruitless worry.

Once a decision is carefully reached we should get busy carrying out our decisions and should not bother about all the anxieties that are about to come. When we, or any of our colleagues or associates, are about to worry about a problem, we must write it out and think of the following questions: Instead of worrying about what people say, why not spend time trying to accomplish something they may admire. What if we just acted like everything was easy? How would your life be different if we stopped worrying about things we can't control and started focusing on the things we can? Let today be the day. We must free ourselves from fruitless worry, seize the day and take effective action on things we can change thus we would see that our lives changes for the betterment and we are on the right path of a sweet, good and happy living.

LEAVE WORRIES NOW
BE HAPPY ENJOY LIFE
CHAPTER 36

LIFE IS TO LIVE HAPPILY

Annalise sweet good and happy living and stop worrying over petty matters. Generate sweet living and generate good thoughts. Don't wait around or expect others to create happiness that is entirely yours to make. Whatever your goal is, do whatever you have to do to get it, always keep yourself to be a happy person. Why worry about the future. Just imagine as to what if we just acted like everything was easy and there was nothing very serious about it to come in future. Worry often gives a small thing a big shadow and its surrounding do frightened with more scary things with the result we do not tend to have a happy life or a sweet and happing living.

Make yourself aware of what's possible in this world.

Worrying will carry tomorrow's load with today's strength. Worry will not empty tomorrow of its sorrows, but it tends to empty today of its power and strength. Worries make you to move into tomorrow ahead of time. Half the worry in the world is caused by people trying to make decisions before they have sufficient knowledge on which to base a decision. Their negative thoughts pressurise them to be away from the positivity in their lives as they fail and do not analysis on positive and they fail to lead a happy life or sweet life.

Why worry about tomorrow;

Concentrate on today happening as for tomorrow will worry about itself. Each day has its own worries and troubles. Always think that you are a happy man. If there is not any solution to the some problem then do not waste time worrying about it. And if there is a solution to the problem then why waste time worrying about it. Act fast be happy generate positive happiness worries will automatically vanish in the air and you are sure to lead a sweet life and happy life.

The first step to good and happy is by way of creating good and happy thoughts in your minds.

Focus your imagination and make efforts on becoming new positive person. Create happiness in you. Divert your mind to good thoughts. It is much easier to bring about change if you just put your mind to it and change your thoughts into a much more positive direction. We know that it is difficult for us to control things that happen in our lives, but we can, with some effort, control what we think or do in our lives. Positive thoughts will make our imagination livelier and we would be able to lead our lives happily without many worries.

The second good step is to have the company of good and positive living friends.

Appreciate the people in your life who have stood by you through thick and thin. Count their support and analyses the happiness in them which will help you to lead a much happier life.

Good friends help each other in the days of crises and through both the good and bad times. Keep yourself busy and surround yourself with good friends, who always think positive. Feel positive about them and feel lucky to have them in your company. Share positive thoughts with them. Tell them to be happy and to lead a sweet good and happy life.

The third step is to focus your imagination on happy things in life by giving a good smile.

The easiest way is feeling happy. Many theories have revealed that happiness can lift one's mood and can divert your mind to sweet living. We may also share positivity with others by flashing them with a brilliant and good smile. Positive and sweet talks are the rewards of good and happy thoughts it generates more happiness. Dejection, disappointments and depression, however, have consequences that could ruin our health, and life. We must divert their minds to focus to the imagination of good and happy life If something bad or good is to happen it is sure to happen, whether we are sad or unhappy or depressed. Let us put our energy into today and stop worrying about the future and past. We should not foresee trouble, or worry about what may never happen as past is dead and gone forever and future is uncertain and yet to come. Be your unabashed self in all the best ways that you can.

The basic facts we should know about happiness.

The basic techniques to analyze happiness and how to break the unhappy habits before it breaks us.

These are the simple ways where we can concentrate and get rid of unhappy thoughts. Annalise unhappiness to see and get the reasons and facts as to why we worry. To avoid reoccurrence of worries, concentrate on prayers as prayers are the best source of remedies of the prevailing worries. The more you pray, the less you'll panic. The more you worship, the less you worry. There is nothing that wastes the body like worry, and anyone who has any faith in God should need not to worry about anything whatsoever is to happen in future. This will ease our way to a sweet good and happy living.

What do we think about happy thoughts?

The feeling of happiness   is within us. It is said that sweet good and happy living is purely our own matter and it has nothing to do with our external circumstances. There is something very special within us which keeps us happy and there is something very unpleasant within us which keeps unhappy. Yes quite true it is the positiveness within us that make and creates happiness within us. Happy living through positivity is nothing more than that of living a normal life free from undue pressures, problems and tensions. If we want to live a happy life then we need to get rid of the negativity and we must try to avoid all the unpleasant things within us which makes us unhappy.

Negative approach always complicates the problems and increases unhappiness.

Most of us do the fatal mistake of looking outwards for happiness rather than looking inwards. Be happy, be strong, be bold and be courageous every day.

Even if we are having a bad day, think of some good things that may come our way, either later that day, tomorrow, next week, month, or next moment.

Simply making castles in the air won't solve our problems.

When everything seems to be beyond our control, it's almost too easy for us to slip into the grasp of unhappiness. To avoid unhappiness we must strive to abolish this sort of thinking through the power of thinking positively. We ought to know the basic fundamental of analyzing happiness. Worries and unhappiness create unnecessary thoughts and these are caused by people going in for unwanted decisions, fore hand not even knowing as to when a good decision is made and not even having sufficient knowledge about it. We must first study and after carefully weighing all the facts than only come to a powerful decision. Simply making castles in the air won't solve our problems but add more to our vows and unhappiness which may even lead us to unhappy life. Anxiety and worry can go hand in hand. When anxiety grabs the mind, it is self-perpetuating. Your mind gets clogged with numerous buts and ifs. Do not worry about your life.

Negativity and worries are repetitive thoughts

Negativity and worries are repetitive thoughts associated with feelings of anxiety in anticipation of some negative future event. Worries and anxious feelings lead to disasters and make our lives unhappy.

If we know that our circumstances are beyond our control or power we need to change them or revise them to our liking. We must try to put a stop-less order on our worries. We must be careful and we need not permit little things which become insects of our lives to ruin our happiness. Co-operate with the inevitable. Decide just how much anxiety a thing may be worth and refuse to give in anymore. All the happiness is not given in one go it comes slowly and slowly. We must pay special attention to remain happy and be happy. Keep ourselves happy, treat our worried thoughts as valuable signals to a sweet living good and happy living.

The utmost cause of unhappiness is your state of depression.

Unhappiness is not there to motivate information gathering or problem-solving. In fact it is depression that constructs the future of unhappiness. Depression is inertia. That's the thing about depression: depression is so insidious, and it compounds daily, and it's impossible to ever see the end of it.

Keep yourself happy

Depressed people think they know themselves, but maybe they only know depression. There are no hopeless than this to get depressed create unhappiness in our minds and become unhappy all the time. Our attitude towards suffering and depression becomes very important because it can affect how we cope with suffering when it arises. Depression is nourished by a lifetime of grieved and unforgiven causes.

Another factor to remain unhappy is worrying about unwanted and useless things. Worry is a misuse of the imagination. To keep yourself happy, treat your worried thoughts as most unwanted assets. These are the fundamental facts you should be familiar about worries. A huge factor to stay happy is to cater your worries around, an important relationship in your life and pay special attention sustaining positive relationships. Make your mind firm and do come to a positive decision and not allow the worries to un-ease the power your mind and soul that can cause unhappiness in you.

We must free ourselves from fruitless worry.

Once a decision is carefully reached we should get busy carrying out our decisions and should not bother about all the anxieties that are about to come. When we, or any of our colleagues or associates, are about to worry about a problem, we must write it out and think of the following questions: Instead of worrying about what people say, why not spend time trying to accomplish something they may admire. What if we just acted like everything was easy? How would your life be different if we stopped worrying about things we can't control and started focusing on the things we can? Let today be the day. We must free ourselves from fruitless worry, seize the day and take effective action on things we can change thus we would see that our lives changes for the betterment and we are on the right path of a sweet, good and happy living.

LEAVE WORRIES NOW
BE HAPPY ENJOY LIFE

CHAPTER 37

WHY WORRY AND UNHAPPY LIVING

We must have to learn to swim out of the sorrows.

It is a common fact that no one in this world is free of obstacles or difficulties. If all the openings of happiness are shut for us and we have to overcome that and have no way to come out, but to survive lest we must have to learn to swim out of the sorrows because this is what is called life and sorrow free living. There are lot more examples and in many other situations, where we will find that how we could have faced and fought with our sorrows and difficulties of life when there was no hope left in our lives.

Fighting for survival is what is needed at odd intervals.

Once we start thinking more positively and happily, we will realize that we had to reinforce these thoughts and behaviors within ourselves so that we could stick to it. As with any sort of training, the more we practice, the better we get to be positive.

The best and easiest way to do this is to be positive when it comes to who we are. We need to speak to ourselves that we are awesome. And we have done a good job at work thus creating positivity within us. We need to be honest with ourselves, and we need to do our best to look for the good.

And, whatever we do, we must not focus on the negative but focus as to how we can become happy by discarding all negative thoughts and have the feeling to remain happy and gay. It is alright not to like everything about ourselves, but don't focus on what we don't like. We have all the positive attributes, and it's up to us to remind ourselves of them every day in order to make us to live happily in our lives.

Life is such a special gift of Almighty so always be happy

Life is such a special gift of Almighty and it is not gifted by Him to use it the way we like or love to. The actual path shown by Him needs to be followed by us for us to reach the peak of betterment every moment. We need to have some happy attitude to look at it comfortably but at the same time having a positive mental attitude does not mean banishing all negative thoughts and people from your life. The same is true with thoughts. When we go to field with negative thoughts, we banish one and another one arises. Therefore creation of positivity and creation of happiness in life is utmost necessary to enjoy the special gift of God to us.

Do not create unnecessary worries.

If we try to change the way we look, talk and behave just to please others, and show our pride we will gradually become such a person that we ourselves won't recognize each other and would start and create unnecessary worries within us and our surrounding without being positive and will not start to live happily.

Thus we must behave in such a manner so as not to create unnecessary worries in our thoughts and mind. We ought to stop worrying over unnecessary things be positive and live without fear happily. We need to understand that what people think of us is their concern, and not ours. If they think about us to be, too reticent or proud, it's really not our business. If every time we happen to meet some new fellows, we may wonder and imagine as what they think of us, and with this feeling in us we will never be able to live a trouble-free and hassle free life. We are bound to fall into the trap of unnecessary worries denying us the startup of new and the happy living life. We would not be able to lead a sweet good and happy life. The main reason is that we must think rationally. Is it in our hands or can we control what others think about us? Simply we need to ignore them. If we cannot, and live our lives the way we want to and find the ways to leave worries aside and start living a happy life. Let us make our way to happy living.

Happy Living with Positive Attitudes.

Positive thinking is not about putting on a pair of rose-colored glasses and ignoring all the negative things you will encounter in life. That approach can be just as devastating as ignoring the positive and only focusing on the negative. Balance, with a healthy dose of realism, is the key. It is a well-known fact that attitude decides how a natives or persons copes up with the day to day events of life. Attitude is what a influence a person's reaction to a situation in life is. It sets the emotional undertone for a person to his likes or dislikes a situation even before he is acquainted with it.

Positive attitude is a quality that is second to none in a human being. Though we attach so much importance to this attitude, as we grow into teenage and adult years we find ourselves becoming ungrateful or taking things for granted. We lose touch with the very same qualities that we instill in our children. We take for granted our life, our health, our families, the people in our lives, the things that our loved ones do for us to make our lives easier and things that we possess.

The positive attitude and happy face speaks a lot about a person.

It denotes about changing negative happiness and making positive thinking and living a positive attitude a good habit. Thinking positively and a positive attitude help us to appreciate and value ourselves, our potential and all that we have. It ensures that we do not take our abilities for granted. It makes us look at ourselves as special people with a special set of abilities and potential. It banishes the feelings of inadequacy and insecurity that arises from unfair comparisons with others. It helps us to appreciate people for who they are and not magnify what they are not and their little flaws. It drives away prejudice and makes us approach life with an open mind. It predisposes us to react to the daily events of life in a positive manner and help us to look at the brighter side of life. Make us optimistic. It gives hope and helps us look forward to life with anticipation and makes us to live happily. We need to know that positive thinking takes the focus away from what we don't have, to appreciating and making good use of what we have.

It is closely connected to our emotional wellbeing and happiness. We feel loved and at peace with ourselves for a major part of our lives when we make this attitude ours. This adds and helps us to get rid of greed, amenity, bitterness, jealousy, and promotes a healthy and nurturing attitude towards others, which in turn gets reciprocated and we feel the sense of healthy living. We attach so much importance to this attitude of gratitude that when our children fail to thank someone, we insist that they do it. That is what is needed to be avoided from time to time. We expect this in return from others when we help them or give them a gift. We call a person discourteous and rude when they do not say thank us in return. On the face of it we ought to know that a positive is not an attitude of being satisfied and content, that you never want to do anything, anymore. This is an attitude that makes you feel good about who you are, what you do, and what your potentials are. This attitude impels you to utilize all that you are endowed with as a person, to achieve the highest possible goals. When we have this attitude, we are able to work without any external pressure to perform but there is sufficient pressure and motivation from within.

The possessing of happy living is like any other habit.

The possessing of happy living is like any other habit, so you need to follow the routine of habit formation here as well. You will win new friends and admirers without having to impress them or conform to the pressure of doing things their way. You will be bubbling with life. You will be rearing to go and accomplish all you can with your new found confidence.

The best part of adopting the 'happy living" is a positive attitude of gratitude is that, you will be able to enjoy the smallest pleasures of nature with a heightened sense of satisfaction and awe. You can see and watch a beautiful flower and carry that joy in your mind for future enjoyment with a clear positive habit. You can go back to work freshen and can use it as an object to meditate on when you feel stressed. You can converge to form of happy living with this habit of positive and sweet living. You need to remember that the possession of happy living is like any other habit and one need not practice so hard to get it .Let us be clear that a positive is not an attitude of being satisfied and content, that we never want to do anything, anymore. This is an attitude that makes you feel good about who you are, what you do, and what your potentials are. This attitude impels you to utilize all that you are endowed with as a person, to achieve the highest possible goals. When we have this attitude, we are able to work without any external pressure to perform but there is sufficient pressure and motivation from within. The habit of happy living is like any other habit, so we need to follow the routine of habit formation here as well.

Keeping our dreams and hope alive our success and happiness.

We should not forget that happiness in life comes through the doors of positive thoughts; we need to have them first. If one door happen to close, another opens, in the event only when we are confident and optimistic. We have so many reasons to cry and at the same time plenty of reasons to smile as well.

Similarly, happiness does not stand for anything, but is on our way of thinking that how do we keep ourselves happy in life. Failure and disappointment are part of our life. The only thing is that we need to face and solve the problem is by keeping our dreams and hope alive be it a reason that success and happiness will come our way again. The experience has taught us that we should buy some strength, hope and positivity from our loved ones to help ourselves in such a situation rather than surrendering as life is a precious gift of God and is equipped with full of joy and happiness if we help ourselves in these critical moments we can live with considerable optimism.

Life is there, where there is hope.

What if when everything goes wrong and all the doors of happiness are closed our live becomes a silent. It is a quite common and we are aware of a marvelous proverb that Life itself is a stage and we all are the performers, performing different acts assigned to us by our almighty power. We should always remember that, "Life is there, where there is hope". That single thing that remains in our hands is to find out ways to know how to overcome these worries of our life at that very moment when all doors are closed for us which means that whatever situation is there, we must not give up hope. We must fight because there have been always a chance that with good faith and hard work we can turn the odds in our favor. It is often said that it is very easy to advice but when it comes to us, things go out of our control and we fail to suggest a way out for ourselves. We fall into the trap of unnecessary worries and elope ourselves with negative thoughts.

We feel better when somebody else is facing some difficulty but when it comes to us we fail to gather that faith, will power and the words of strength. When the power of will is at the worst and each one of us knows that the one who is gone never comes back. Neither a thousands of words would not be enough to bring him back nor a million tears, because each and every moment, eyes would only shed tears , mind would remain tensed and we would be simply surrounded by worries and the life seems to have been vanished. Life is ever expanding, contraction is death. As commonly said by big saints that the self- seeking man who is looking after his personal comforts and leading a lazy life for himself there would be no room for him even in the hell and he simply have lost the power of his will.We are quite aware of the fact that faith in oneself is the history of a man and that faith calls the quality of superiority within a person. One cannot do anything without it. We fail only when we do not try very hard to achieve the power and faith within us. As soon as we lose faith, death comes in our way and we are surrounds by all the evils and stupid worries of the world.

The secret of every successful man is to have, good confidence, faith and strength

The secret and history of every successful man is to have, good confidence, faith and strength behind him and that remain the right cause of his single success in life. Unselfishness plays a very vital role in his life. He may not have been perfectly unselfish, yet he was tending towards it. If he had been perfectly unselfish, he would have been as great a success.

The degree of unselfishness marks the degree of success everywhere and he leads to be successful man without fear worries and selfishness. There are quite a number of reasons to believe that for a successful and happy life the mystery surrounding it lies in our interests, and good memory which is the basis of our interest, power of desire and aim, keeping ourselves smiling and the doubt free character which is the foremost important reason for a successful and happy life. If we possess one solid unselfish and doubt free character within ourselves we would be quite happy and successful.

The love for God and worshipping.

The love for God and worshipping God adds to one common thing the immense faith in Him. There may be different beliefs and ways to worship God in different communities, places and religions, but one thing remains the same and that is the Love of God for all of us. Our world is full of odds and evens, happiness and sorrows, fulfilment and emptiness. And these are all created by the Almighty. However, the most beautiful Gift of God, is a Human, which is such a mystery driven by Him which could hardly be defined or explained in depth.

The secret of successful and happy life lies in keeping ourselves smiling.

The secret of successful and happy life lies in keeping ourselves smiling and the character which is the foremost important reason that lies within us. Do not be curious about anything, but in everything, by prayer and petition, with thanksgiving, present your requests to God.

Whenever your mind is tempted to jump the fence and start to worry, say this verse aloud or to yourself. You may even have to repeat it over and over again.

Steps for a successful and happy life.

Being a positive thinker is not about ignoring reality in favor of aspirational thoughts. It is more about taking a proactive approach to your life. Instead of feeling hopeless or overwhelmed, positive thinking allows you to tackle life's challenges by looking for effective ways to resolve conflict and come up with creative solutions to problems.

Life is not a bed of roses.

Life is a battle field and not a bed of roses as every man on earth has to struggle very hard in making his life happy. If aim of our life is to stay happy and let others to be happy, we will be happy and remembered by all. But no one will actually remember us for the wealth we have gained, or success we have achieved. If we have no aim in life, we would not be able to lead and happy life. Living with no purpose in life is just like a feather moving towards the wind. Both career and purpose are different issues but it is equally important to understand the value of these things which would ultimately add spicy flavor to your living. Innovation at work place is what it necessary is how well we judge our work, how good we like and enjoy it. If we take our work as a stiff challenge and as learning everyday then we would start loving it and giving our best. However, if we just work for the sake of then nothing is realized and we do not remain happy in life.

We should not aim to have negative thoughts at all.

Now let's us imagine that we are not feeling at our best today, and we are having thoughts that could be classified as negative. We shouldn't be thinking such negative thoughts. We don't like the negative thoughts. We ought to know that negative thoughts are stressful, demoralizing and depressing. We shouldn't aim to have negative thoughts at all. Often we feel uncomfortable because we think we have to say or do something in response to another person's words. When we find ourselves thinking this way, it helps enormously to take a few moments to check inside and notice what we are feeling. Negative thoughts destroy our happy livings. We ought to discard all these negative thought and act to live in a more positive atmosphere rather than living in a negative world where we can never find a happy living.

LEAVE WORRIES NOW
BE HAPPY ENJOY LIFE

CHAPTER 38

STEPS FOR A SUCCESSFUL AND HAPPY LIFE

It might not be easy, but the positive impact it will have on our mental, emotional, and physical health will be well-worth it .At time we may think that there is no road is left for us from where we can achieve the happiness of our lives. We may also feel that life has become terrible for us to live and we are carrying new hope that someone would come to rescue us. There may be chances that someone who was there with us before might have held on to us when we were on the dark side of the life.

Life itself is a stage and we all are the performers.

What if when everything goes wrong and all the doors of happiness are closed our live becomes a silent. It is a quite common and we are aware of a marvelous proverb that Life itself is a stage and we all are the performers, performing different acts assigned to us by our almighty power. We should not forget as to what is in our possession, if it is to fulfill our duties towards our responsibility and do whatever is correct and is allowed by us in our life? We should not forget that happiness in life comes through the doors of positive thoughts; we need to have them first. If one door happen to close, another opens, in the event only when we are confident and optimistic.

We have so many reasons to cry and at the same time plenty of reasons to smile as well. Similarly, happiness does not stand for anything, but is on our way of thinking that how do we keep ourselves happy in life. Failure and disappointment are part of our life. The only thing is that we need to face and solve the problem is by keeping our dreams and hope alive be it a reason that success and happiness will come our way again.

Smiling and the doubt free character which is the foremost important reason for a successful and happy life.

There are quite a number of reasons to believe that for a successful and happy life the mystery surrounding it lies in our interests, and good memory which is the basis of our interest, power of desire and aim, keeping ourselves smiling and the doubt free character which is the foremost important reason for a successful and happy life. If we possess one solid unselfish and doubt free character within ourselves we would be quite happy and successful. The experience has taught us that we should buy some strength, hope and positivity from our loved ones to help ourselves in such a situation rather than surrendering as life is a precious gift of God and is equipped with full of joy and happiness if we help ourselves in these critical moments we can live with considerable optimism. Now let's us imagine that we are not feeling at our best today, and we are having thoughts that could be classified as negative. We shouldn't be thinking such negative thoughts. We don't like the negative thoughts. We ought to know that negative thoughts are stressful, demoralizing and depressing.

We shouldn't aim to have negative thoughts at all. Often we feel uncomfortable because we think we have to say or do something in response to another person's words. When we find ourselves thinking this way, it helps enormously to take a few moments to check inside and notice what we are feeling. We are deeply depressed that negativity has governed us and has taken a deep root in our minds. So, let's imagine that you have chosen to focus on your negative thinking with regards to school.

Evaluating thoughts can generate happiness within us.

The next step is to spend a little bit of time each day evaluating your own thoughts. When you find yourself thinking critical thoughts about yourself, take a moment to pause and reflect. While you might be upset about getting a bad grade on an exam, is berating yourself really the best approach? Is there any way to put a positive spin on the situation? While you might not have done well on this exam, at least you have a better indication of how to structure your study time for the next big test. However, despite of all these good thoughts which are embodied to us by the almighty fail to revive these unwanted circumstances that lead us to sorrow and difficulties and a situation where we do not know what is correct and good for us and what is wrong for us.

Life is there, where there is hope.

We should always remember that, "Life is there, where there is hope".

That single thing that remains in our hands is to find out ways to know how to overcome these worries of our life at that very moment when all doors are closed for us which means that whatever situation is there, we must not give up hope. We must fight because there have been always a chance that with good faith and hard work we can turn the odds in our favor. It is often said that it is very easy to advice but when it comes to us, things go out of our control and we fail to suggest a way out for ourselves.

Happy living allows us to tackle life's challenges

We fall into the trap of unnecessary worries and elope ourselves with negative thoughts. We feel better when somebody else is facing some difficulty but when it comes to us we fail to gather that faith, will power and the words of strength. Being a positive thinker is not about ignoring reality in favor of aspirational thoughts. It is more about taking a proactive approach to our lives. Instead of feeling hopeless or overwhelmed, positive thinking allows us to tackle life's challenges by looking for effective ways to resolve conflict and come up with creative solutions to problems. It might not be easy, but the positive impact it will have on our mental, emotional, and physical health will be well-worth it. It takes practice; lots of practice. This is not a step-by-step process that we can complete and be done with. Instead, it involves a lifelong commitment to looking inside ourselves and being willing to challenge negative thoughts and make positive changes. It is a common fact that no one in this world is free of obstacles or difficulties.

If all the openings of happiness are shut for us and we have to overcome that and have no way to come out, but to survive lest we must have to learn to swim out of the sorrows because this is what is called life and sorrow free living. There are lot more examples and in many other situations, where we will find that how we could have faced and fought with our sorrows and difficulties of life when there was no hope left in our lives. As commonly said by big saints that the self- seeking man who is looking after his personal comforts and leading a lazy life for himself there would be no room for him even in the hell and he simply have lost the power of his will and he cannot lead a happy life.

The secret of every successful man is to have, good confidence

The secret of every successful man is to have, good confidence, faith and strength behind him and that remain the right cause of his single success in life. Unselfishness plays a very vital role in his life. He may not have been perfectly unselfish, yet he was tending towards it. If he had been perfectly unselfish, he would have been as great a success. The degree of unselfishness marks the degree of success everywhere and he leads to be successful man without fear worries and selfishness. Therefore creation of positivity in life is utmost necessary to enjoy the special gift of God to us. The love for God and worshipping God adds to one common thing the immense faith in Him. There may be different beliefs and ways to worship God in different communities, places and religions, but one thing remains the same and that is the Love of God for all of us.

Our world is full of odds and evens, happiness and sorrows, fulfilment and emptiness. And these are all created by the Almighty. However, the most beautiful Gift of God, is Human, which is such a mystery driven by Him which could hardly be defined or explained in depth.

If aim of our life is to stay happy and let others to be happy, we will be happy and remembered by all.

We know that life cannot be foreseen. Life is not a bed of roses. Life is a battle field and not a bed of roses as every man on earth has to struggle very hard in making his life happy. But no one will actually remember us for the wealth we have gained, or success we have achieved until and unless we do not live a happy life. Life is such a special gift of Almighty and it is not gifted by Him to use it the way we like or love to. The actual path shown by Him needs to be followed by us for us to reach the peak of betterment every moment. We need to have some positive attitude to look at it comfortably but at the same time having a positive mental attitude does not mean banishing all negative thoughts and people from your life. We need to believe that a positive attitude is a choice. This step is hard to take. People are either positive or negative. They tend to blame their negativity on all kinds of outside forces fate, experiences, parents, relationship, but never really stopped to think that they could choose to be positive. Piercing ourselves that positivity is a choice has been one of the greatest things we have ever done for ourselves. Now when we find ourselves in a bad situation, we know that it's up to us to find the good, to be positive regardless of what's happening around us.

We should no longer point fingers and place blame to anyone else. We need to realize that everything happens how it happens, and it's up to us to choose how we want to feel about it. We need to be in control of our attitude, and no one can take that away this from us. If we want to live a positive, joyful and happy life, we must not be surrounded by negative people who don't encourage our happiness. As a negative person, we ought to get attracted too negative people only. Only when we decide to make the change to live a more positive life, we have to get rid of our lives of the most negative influences in it. We are quite aware of the fact that no one is perfect and perfection isn't the goal when it comes to positivity but there were people in our lives who were consistently negative, who constantly bring us down, we need to stop spending so much time with them.

We can very well imagine, it is not easy for us to get away from these negative people.

It can hurt us to keep distance from people even when you know they aren't good for us and for our current lifestyle. In addition to removing negative influences from them, we also have to get rid of some of our own negative behaviors, such as the drug and alcohol abuse. We need to take some concrete steps and examine which behaviors are good for us and which were not harmful. What we need is to learn to focus on the positive things, such as working on positive activities and cultivating new, positive relationships. We must let go of the negative ones.

This process may be not easy to live a positive life when negative people and behaviors continually pull us down. In every situation or in every person there is something good.

Anything good and bad is learning experience.

Most of the time it's not easy to find the positive qualities but we have to look hard to discover positivity in them. Now, when we are faced with a difficult or challenging situation, we need to think and talk to ourselves and console our mind, no matter how terrible the situation might seem, we can always find something good if we take the time to think about it. It is quite obvious that anything good and bad is learning experience so, at the very least, we must learn from bad experiences.

However, there's usually even more to it than that. If you really take some time to have a look at it, we would find something good, something genuinely positive, about every person or situation. Not only do we need to be happy with ourselves for this multiple action to take effect, but we also need to be more positive and happy with others. We have to share our wealth of happiness with the people of the world. The best way is to be nice with other people, no matter what. Tell them that they look nice today. Appreciate their job and tell them that have done a great job on that assignment. Be happy and tell your elder or your kids how much you love them and how great they are. When someone is feeling down, do what we need to do is to cheer him or her up. Do send them gifts nice flower and glow them with nice notes. By doing this we will not make ourselves happy but in turn give and generate happiness for others too.

At times we may suffer from chronic depression, though we know how good things look on to others life cannot be worse for us. Let's imagine how to deal when life leaves a great big steaming pile at our doorstep. Lest we need to remember that external factors can be dealt with by taking positive and happy steps to repair or at least address the root of the problem as best as we can. Whatever may be the primary cause of the problem, that cause must be examined first? What is required is that we never wanted to see the good in ourselves and, therefore, didn't want to see it in others also. We must not be critical and condescending rather we must be encouraging and supportive. We should not try to treat others as we would like to be treated, but also try to consider how we would like to be treated. The world likes to appreciate positivity, and the more we share it with others, the more we would be practicing it your own lives. When we start feeling like the idea of not being a happy person we need to remind ourselves that all it takes is one tiny step in the right direction to move towards a more happy life.

Share your happy thoughts with others

We have to believe in ourselves and remember the most important lesson of all is a happy outlook and that is a choice that we can always make. The power of remaining happy, whatever the situation, can never be underestimated. We are all here for a short duration, but is it worth it to spend any of that time in a any angry or being negative? That need to sort out in mind and soul and thus must share our happy thoughts with others.

The real test of any one is to remain happy whenever some challenges become difficult. Remaining happy keeps our mind in the right state of balance and often opens resolutions to the problems at hand. Negativity is contagious and spreads like fire. It not only does its affect anyone, but it spreads to everyone who ever comes in contact with it or whoever they interact with. When only the negative perspective is in focus, the resolution process is impeded. Eliminating negativity, or rather, being positive is a mindset that can be found at any moment, and which can be turned into a habit. We must throw away the negativity in us and opt for being a very positive person this in turn will make us happy and we would be able to lead a sweet and happy life forever.

LEAVE WORRIES NOW
BE HAPPY ENJOY LIFE

CHAPTER 39

MAKE YOUR WAY TO HAPPY LIVING

The secret of successful and happy life lies in keeping ourselves smiling

We need to learn a lesson from every situation. No matter how difficult the situation may appear. We should recognize the beautiful lessons waiting to be discovered. Sometimes lessons may prove to be expensive and costly, but every problem is a learning experience in disguise. We need to be conscious of our thoughts, especially, when life just isn't going our way. The moment we see that we are diving into frustration, agony, sorrow or low self –esteem we must shift our thoughts, by thinking about something completely different and unrelated. You are essentially trying to cultivate a new habit here, the secret of successful and happy life lies in keeping ourselves smiling and the character which is the foremost important reason that lies within us. Whenever your mind is tempted to jump the fence and start to worry, say this verse aloud or to yourself. You may even have to repeat it over and over again. Am I constantly striving to see the positive in every aspect of my life? Steps for a successful and happy life.

MAKE YOUR WAY TO HAPPY LIVING

We need to believe that a happy living is a matter of our choice. This step is hard to take.

People are either positive or negative. They tend to blame their negativity on all kinds of outside forces fate, experiences, parents, relationship, but never really stopped to think that they could choose to be happy. Piercing ourselves that happiness is a choice has been one of the greatest things we have ever done for ourselves.

Now when we find ourselves in a bad situation, we know that it is up to us to find the good, to be happy regardless of what is happening around us. We should no longer point fingers and place blame to anyone else. We need to realise that everything happens how it happens, and it is up to us to choose how we want to feel about it. We need to be in control of our attitude and happiness, and no one can take that away this from us.

Unhappiness is contagious and spreads like fire.

It not only does its affect anyone, but it spreads to everyone who ever comes in contact with it or whoever they interact with. When only the negative perspective is in focus, the resolution process is impeded. Eliminating unhappiness, or rather, being happy is a mindset that can be found at any moment, and which can be turned into a habit.

If we want to live a happy, joyful life, we must not be surrounded by negative people who don't encourage our happiness. As a negative person, we ought to get attracted to negative people only. Only when we decide to make the change to live a more positive and happy life, we have to get rid of our lives of the most negative influences in it.

We are quite aware of the fact that no one is perfect and perfection is not the goal when it comes to positivity but there were people in our lives who were consistently negative, who constantly bring us down, we need to stop spending so much time with them. We can very well imagine, it is not easy for us to get away from these unhappy people. It can hurt us to keep distance from people even when you know they are not good for us and for our current lifestyle. In addition to removing negative influences from them, we also have to get rid of some of our own negative behaviors, such as the drug and alcohol abuse. We need to take some concrete steps and examine which behaviors are good for us and which were not harmful. What we need is to learn to focus on the happy things, such as working on positive activities and cultivating new, positive relationships. We must let go of the negative ones.

This process may be not easy to live a positive life when negative people and behaviors continually pull us down. We need to discard all of them to lead a happy and sweet life. An art of sweet living lies below us we have only to recognize it. The real test of any one is to remain happy whenever some challenges become difficult. Remaining happy keeps our mind in the right state of balance and often opens resolutions to the problems at hand. We must throw away the unhappiness in us and opt for being a very positive person. In every situation or in every person there is something good. Most of the time it's not easy to find the happiness qualities but we have to look hard to discover happiness in them.

Now, when we are faced with a difficult or challenging situation, we need to think and talk to ourselves and console our mind, no matter how terrible the situation might seem, we can always find something good if we take the time to think about it. It is quite obvious that anything good and bad is learning experience so, at the very least, we must learn from bad experiences. However, there is usually even more to it than that. If you really take some time to have a look at it, we would find something good, something genuinely happy, about every person or situation. We must look for sweet living in life

Get Sweet feeling in your life

Once we start thinking more in a happy manner, we will realize that we had to reinforce these thoughts and behaviors within ourselves so that we could stick to it. As with any sort of training, the more we practice, the better we get to be happy.

The best and easiest way to do this is to be happy when it comes to who we are. We need to speak to ourselves that we are awesome. And we have done a good job at work thus creating happiness within us. We need to be honest with ourselves, and we need to do our best to look for the good. And, whatever we do, we must not focus on the negative. It is alright not to like everything about ourselves, but don not focus on what we do not like. We have all to get the sweet feeling in our lives, and it is up to us to remind ourselves of them every day.

Share sweet and happy thoughts

Not only do we need to be happy with ourselves for this multiple action to take effect, but we need to be happier with others too. We have to share our wealth of happiness with the people of the world. The best way is to be nice with other people and to make them happy, no matter what the matter is. Tell them that they look nice today. What is required is that we never wanted to see the good in ourselves and, therefore, didn't want to see it in others also. We must not be critical and condescending rather we must be encouraging and supportive. We should not try to treat others as we would like to be treated, but also try to consider how we would like to be treated. This will strangle the pattern of self-pity, mind-created imaginations, and negative downward stairs. Really what makes us different from other mammals is our ability to control our thoughts and think for ourselves happiness and shift our unhappy thoughts to a happy feelings and to happy living. We may have made mistakes, but now we can accept it and continue, knowing that we will make a different decision in the future. If we understand this it can be appreciative for the experience. We cannot be both angry and grateful at the same time. We should start counting the blessings and miracles in our lives and if we start exploring for them and we would find more happiness in doing so.

Feeling good about ourselves and showing self-confidence.

Feeling good about ourselves and showing self-confidence boosts our skills potential and capabilities in any areas of work and supports us to become happier.

We need to shift our thoughts from being a unhappy person to more strong and positive man. Also keeping in mind that pushing things to the limit and going beyond what we think is possible for us to get to the next step of being happy. It becomes another key to achieving what we really want to do. We only want happiness and want to lead a happy life. Even if it may even be relationships and we are finding it difficult to meet someone where we are actually interested in, we need not wait because it usually doesn't come to us by own, we must stand up to get help from any learned fellow. One of the most important things while doing all of this is to be happy about what we are doing, thus we ought to have a successful goal setting our lifestyle with a happy attitude. We may or may not be able to solve the problem of unhappiness that lies within us, but at least knowing that we are taking positive steps that can help us improve our happiness. It will not be easy, of course, for us and it may be like suffering a chronic disease thus we must balance ourselves as "being happy" with an understanding that the reality is, it is going to be an ongoing battle for our own survival. Depression will undermine even the strongest of wills, need help to maintain or at least be reminded of a happy outlook and happiness that is prevailing within us .Counseling, psychotherapy, and the right combination of medication will play a crucial role in helping to keep us from sinking into that very dark place that is the essence of depression and unhappiness. Be patient, but don't look for miracles. It may be that we will need the help of professionals throughout our lives to maintain a generally even keel. If one could "will away" depression, there would be no need of doctors or drugs.

What we can do is understand why we feel like we do, and explain to our counselors that we wish it were that easy, and that we appreciate our concern towards being happy persons. Shifting our thoughts enables us to the right path of our happiness and thinking in its direction of positivity can make us to lead a very happy life.

LEAVE WORRIES NOW
BE HAPPY ENJOY LIFE

CHAPTER 40

LOOK FOR A SWEET LIVING IN LIFE

Thought which are provoking our mind, about the uncertainties and the negativities, as to what will happen tomorrow. Worries that are prevailing in our minds are repetitive thoughts associated with feelings of anxiety in anticipation of some negative future event. Whether the worries are about financial crisis, family problems, work, health or any topic of concern, the anxious feelings produced and sustained by the imaginary thoughts which always distinctly appear to be unpleasant. Positive

Thinking leads us to a happy life one must not forgot the life is what we make it, so let us make it a happy one!

Don't worry on things that may not happen, life is too short to worry too much. Smile and be happy. Make yourself to be positive person. Keep smiling in the sunlight. Imagine every day to be a positive day and the last of a life surrounded with hopes, the hours that come unexpectedly will be much the more grateful. The mind that is anxious about future events is miserable. Present fears are less than horrible imaginings. Positive thinking is sure to ward of every odd imagination and sure to make you a happy person. Happy living actually means approaching life's challenges with a positive outlook.

It does not necessarily mean avoiding or ignoring the bad things; instead, it involves making the most of potentially bad situations, trying to see the best in other people, and viewing yourself and your abilities in a positive light.Happy living centers on such things as a belief in abilities, a positive approach to challenges, and trying to make the most of bad situations. Bad things will happen. Sometimes you will be disappointed or hurt by the actions of others. This does not mean that the world is out to get you or that all people will let you down. Instead, happy living will look at the situation realistically, search for ways that they can improve the situation, and try to learn from their experiences .Happy living brings good cheer, remembering that the misfortunes hardest to bear are those that never happen, focus on the positive aspects of lives, rather than on the negative setbacks. Let us not waste our lives in doubts and fears. It is not work that kills us, it is worry and the negative thinking. Work is healthy; but worry is rust upon the blade. It is not movement that destroys the machinery, but friction. We need to forget the most disturbing negative thinking in our lives and opt for the positive attitude by following the principles of happy living. Not only can happy living impact our ability to cope with stress and our immunity, it also has an impact on our overall well-being. Our success lies only in our happy living. Look to be happy think in positive terms and think as if the unhappiness is not there at lot and God has given us this precious life to enjoy to our fullest all the fruits of happiness of our lives. Happy living and good living is definitely an "Art of Sweet Living".

LEAVE WORRIES NOW
BE HAPPY ENJOY LIFE

CHAPTER 41

LEAD A TENSION FREE AND HAPPY LIFE

It is often said that mindfulness meditation helps people to develop the skill of being detached and aware. As a result we can become aware of these core irrational beliefs about self, others, and the world without activating self-destructive survival behaviors driven by high stress. We ought to know the simple ways to get people into using mindfulness meditation.. A little stress to keep us energized motivated and hanging out with the people that are doing healthy things. Having a stable relationship these all the primarily things we ought to gather within ourselves. We have to be on the lookout for a possible date with someone. We may even join special groups or clubs of people within our age bracket and who share the same interest. Join church events as well. Try new activities. By expanding our horizon, we will get to know more people who can be a potential date of having a good company. Let us keep life simple. Many of us are always over looking for the most complicated way of doing things in life. We can make our lives to be more simple just take a walk through the park, or a quiet evening with the family. We need not clutter our lives with unnecessary decisions by making everything complicated and complex why not try to keep it simple. Why not practice to be satisfied. Many people don't know how to be satisfied with what life gives them. They are so busy wanting more that they squander what life has already given them. Always urging for more and demanding to have everything making themselves and lives more complicated. Why not practice to be more satisfied we need most.

What we need to beware is of indecision. Life is not that easy at times we have to make tough choices. Never put off a decision that we can make on the day. At times we may miss some of the best and most exciting opportunities in the world because we were indecisive. People who are successful people do not fall prey back and forth on decisions. Let us practice cheerfulness and be happy. We have heard it several times before, and we would hear it here again and again – it only takes a few seconds to smile! We need not be surprised as to how well being cheerful to others can spread like wildfire and make us happy. We live in a society where often glumness is the ruled. A simple smile or kind word can spread through our culture like a fire – not only will we feel better, but those who interact with us will also feel better and best. Therefore why we should not practice cheerfulness and make ourselves happy. How about if we learn to like people and make ourselves happy. We don't have to love everyone we meet; we simply need to learn to like people – especially those who are different than us. Often we may not agree with everything what they do, or maybe with all of their beliefs, but by learning to get along with them we will open our mind up to change – a critical trait that is absolutely necessary in world of today. The most important thing that we must learn is to Live and let live. Is it really our concern what the guy across the other lane wants to do something with his life or wants to share his life with? Why not we learn to live our lives to the fullest and let others live their life to their fullest. We need to bear in mind that we are not above anyone else, and none of us should think we should be allowed to dictate how another person should live and lead their lives. Stop beating over the past happening and let us forgive ourselves. It is simple let us stop beating things that happened in the past – things what we have done or we did not do, and the awful mistakes that we may have made.

Forgiving oneself is a unique skill and only few of us have the ability to accomplish. It's such a shame that we spent a lifetime living in the past and never make it to our full potential in the future. We must forgive ourselves – and just as importantly, forgive others too. It may seem to be a difficult task but if we encourage each other and stop beating over the past we will live a more meaningful, happy and fulfilled life.

LEAVE WORRIES NOW
BE HAPPY ENJOY LIFE

CHAPTER 42

BRING BACK YOUR LIFE TO NORMAL

We need to remember that as we possibly as we can we should make it a point to eat a more balanced, and healthy diet even though we may very little money left with us. We have intake of lot of greens vegetables and with variety of fruit and nuts which are all super healthy food for us, and which are less expensive than meats, cheeses, and processed foods! Their nitrifying value will energize and elevate our body, and knowing this that we are treating ourselves will surely refresh our minds. If we look for rich food rich in vitamins and other useful ingredients which include nuts, soya beans and fatty fish we would get more nutrition value. We must cut back on the caffeine drinks, alcohol. We don't have to quit, but reducing the intake of them will help reduce anxiety and stress from time to time. Exercise is one of health sport that our body needs most. It may be yoga, cross training, or even a simple walking in the park. This helps keeping our body active and will also help to grow our outlook. If we make it hobby we would enjoy the most. Whether its art, photography, music focusing on something other than the worry factor it will give our mind some good atmosphere to breathe off and would generate a good behavior within us. The other refreshing factor is naturally our sleep. We need not be reminded of this. Our body is probably begging us for it when we are in the middle of hard times. We may be drawn to maintain good sleeping habits. Maintain a consistent sleep schedule, but allow yourself some leeway.

If we sleep peacefully let our body get about 8 hours of sleep we get the best results. If you're just starting to have those thoughts, speak to your physician or your therapist. They may prescribe something to help steer you back to the center, emotionally. It may be the act of talking about it is therapeutic enough, but don't assume that. Leave that call to the professionals. Having goals which are set again and again after each one is achieved will give you a mindset or target to strive for which leads to success, with success becomes natural positive attitude. With all costiveness, goals and success builds a higher potential and belief within yourself. Setting realistic goals that you know you can achieve by staying positive is a great beginning to success. Your attitude around your friends, family and public people really tells them who you are, being positive instead of negative makes an excellent first impression on anybody. Positive means to be absolute, clear-cut, definite, forward-looking and expressively firm with a decision. Having a positive attitude toward something means you are willing to commit and do the work without complaint, which leads to goals. You realize that what appears negative today will change tomorrow. Nothing stays the same. Whether you are positive or negative, the situation does not change. So, we mind as well be positive. As with any habit, the habit of remaining positive in all situations takes practice and a commitment to yourself to take control. But start small, start paying attention to your emotions, start by wanting to change. Don't hold onto anything that bothers your mind. It can only hurt your health and it won't help your problems at all. The people that live the longest in this world do not hold grudges or hold onto negative feelings. Visualize your worries on a large chalkboard in your mind. Watch yourself take a big eraser and erase the problems. Every time the thoughts come back into your head, see yourself with the eraser again.

Therefore do not worry about tomorrow, for tomorrow will worry about itself. Each day has enough trouble of its own. Do not anticipate trouble, or worry about what may never happen. Keep in the sunlight. Imagine every day to be the last of a life surrounded with hopes, cares, anger and fear. The hours that come unexpectedly will be much the more grateful. The mind that is anxious about future events is miserable. Present fears are less than horrible imaginings. Let us be of good cheer, remembering that the misfortunes hardest to bear are those that never happen, focus on the positive aspects of their lives, rather than on the negative setbacks. "Feeling confident affects the way we perceive our situations and how we decide to manage them. Don't waste your life in doubts and fears: spend yourself on the work before you, well assured that the right performance of this hour's duties will be the best preparation for the hours or ages that follow it. It is not work that kills men, it is worry. Work is healthy; you can hardly put more on a man than he can bear. But worry is rust upon the blade. It is not movement that destroys the machinery, but friction. Never let life's hardships disturb you ... no one can avoid problems, not even saints or sages. As with any habit, the habit of remaining positive in all situations takes practice and a commitment to yourself to take control. Life is what you make it, so make it a happy one!! Don't worry on things that may not happen, life is too short to worry too much. Smile and be happy

LEAVE WORRIES NOW
BE HAPPY ENJOY LIFE

CHAPTER 43

HAPPINESS AND GOOD LIVING

Annalise sweet good and happy living and stop worrying over petty matters. Generate sweet living and generate good thoughts. Don't wait around or expect others to create happiness that is entirely yours to make. Whatever your goal is, do whatever you have to do to get it, always keep yourself to be a happy person. Why worry about the future. Just imagine as to what if we just acted like everything was easy and there was nothing very serious about it to come in future. Worry often gives a small thing a big shadow and its surrounding do frightened with more scary things with the result we do not tend to have a happy life or a sweet and happing living. Make yourself aware of what's possible in this world.

Worrying will carry tomorrow's load with today's strength. Worry will not empty tomorrow of its sorrows, but it tends to empty today of its power and strength. Worries make you to move into tomorrow ahead of time. Half the worry in the world is caused by people trying to make decisions before they have sufficient knowledge on which to base a decision. Their negative thoughts pressurise them to be away from the positivity in their lives as they fail and do not analysis on positive and they fail to lead a happy life or sweet life.

Concentrate on today's happening

Why worry about tomorrow. Concentrate on today happening as for tomorrow will worry about itself. Each day has its own worries and troubles. Always think that you are a happy man. If there is not any solution to the some problem then do not waste time worrying about it. And if there is a solution to the problem then why waste time worrying about it. Act fast be happy generate positive happiness worries will automatically vanish in the air and you are sure to lead a sweet life and happy life.

The first step to good and happiness is by way of creating good and happy thoughts in your minds.

 Focus your imagination and make efforts on becoming new positive person. Create happiness in you. Divert your mind to good thoughts. It is much easier to bring about change if you just put your mind to it and change your thoughts into a much more positive direction. We know that it is difficult for us to control things that happen in our lives, but we can, with some effort, control what we think or do in our lives. Positive thoughts will make our imagination livelier and we would be able to lead our lives happily without many worries.

The second good step is to have the company of good and positive living friends.

Appreciate the people in your life who have stood by you through thick and thin. Count their support and analyses the happiness in them which will help you to lead a much happier life. Good friends help each other in the days of crises and through both the good and bad times. Keep yourself busy and surround yourself with good friends, who always think positive. Feel positive about them and feel lucky to have them in your company.

Share positive thoughts with them. Tell them to be happy and to lead a sweet good and happy life.

The third step is to focus your imagination on happy things in life by giving a good smile.

The easiest way is feeling happy. Many theories have revealed that happiness can lift one's mood and can divert your mind to sweet living. We may also share positivity with others by flashing them with a brilliant and good smile. Positive and sweet talks are the rewards of good and happy thoughts it generates more happiness. Dejection, disappointments and depression, however, have consequences that could ruin our health, and life. We must divert their minds to focus to the imagination of good and happy life. If something bad or good is to happen it is sure to happen, whether we are sad or unhappy or depressed. Let us put our energy into today and stop worrying about the future and past. We should not foresee trouble, or worry about what may never happen as past is dead and gone forever and future is uncertain and yet to come. Be your unabashed self in all the best ways that you can.

The basic facts we should know about happiness.

The basic techniques to analyze happiness and how to break the unhappy habits before it breaks us. These are the simple ways where we can concentrate and get rid of unhappy thoughts. Annalise unhappiness to see and get the reasons and facts as to why we worry. To avoid reoccurrence of worries, concentrate on prayers as prayers are the best source of remedies of the prevailing worries. The more you pray, the less you'll panic. The more you worship, the less you worry.

There is nothing that wastes the body like worry, and anyone who has any faith in God should need not to worry about anything whatsoever is to happen in future. This will ease our way to a sweet good and happy living.

What do we think about happy thoughts?

The feeling of happiness   is within us.

It is said that sweet good and happy living is purely our own matter and it has nothing to do with our external circumstances. There is something very special within us which keeps us happy and there is something very unpleasant within us which keeps unhappy. Yes quite true it is the positiveness within us that make and creates happiness within us. Happy living through positivity is nothing more than that of living a normal life free from undue pressures, problems and tensions. If we want to live a happy life then we need to get rid of the negativity and we must try to avoid all the unpleasant things within us which makes us unhappy.

Negative approach always complicates the problems and increases unhappiness.

Most of us do the fatal mistake of looking outwards for happiness rather than looking inwards. Be happy, be strong, be bold and be courageous every day. Even if we are having a bad day, think of some good things that may come our way, either later that day, tomorrow, next week, month, or next moment.

Simply making castles in the air won't solve our problems.

When everything seems to be beyond our control, it's almost too easy for us to slip into the grasp of unhappiness.

To avoid unhappiness we must strive to abolish this sort of thinking through the power of thinking positively. We ought to know the basic fundamental of analyzing happiness. Worries and unhappiness create unnecessary thoughts and these are caused by people going in for unwanted decisions, fore hand not even knowing as to when a good decision is made and not even having sufficient knowledge about it. We must first study and after carefully weighing all the facts than only come to a powerful decision. Simply making castles in the air won't solve our problems but add more to our vows and unhappiness which may even lead us to unhappy life. Anxiety and worry can go hand in hand. When anxiety grabs the mind, it is self-perpetuating. Your mind gets clogged with numerous buts and ifs. Do not worry about your life.

Negativity and worries are repetitive thoughts

Negativity and worries are repetitive thoughts associated with feelings of anxiety in anticipation of some negative future event. Worries and anxious feelings lead to disasters and make our lives unhappy. If we know that our circumstances are beyond our control or power we need to change them or revise them to our liking. We must try to put a stop-less order on our worries. We must be careful and we need not permit little things which become insects of our lives to ruin our happiness. Co-operate with the inevitable. Decide just how much anxiety a thing may be worth and refuse to give in anymore. All the happiness is not given in one go it comes slowly and slowly. We must pay special attention to remain happy and be happy. Keep ourselves happy, treat our worried thoughts as valuable signals to a sweet living good and happy living.

The utmost cause of unhappiness is your state of depression. Unhappiness is not there to motivate information gathering or problem-solving. In fact it is depression that constructs the future of unhappiness. Depression is inertia. That's the thing about depression: depression is so insidious, and it compounds daily, and it's impossible to ever see the end of it.

Keep yourself happy

Depressed people think they know themselves, but maybe they only know depression. There are no hopeless than this to get depressed create unhappiness in our minds and become unhappy all the time. Our attitude towards suffering and depression becomes very important because it can affect how we cope with suffering when it arises. Depression is nourished by a lifetime of grieved and unforgiven causes. Another factor to remain unhappy is worrying about unwanted and useless things. Worry is a misuse of the imagination. To keep yourself happy, treat your worried thoughts as most unwanted assets. These are the fundamental facts you should be familiar about worries. A huge factor to stay happy is to cater your worries around, an important relationship in your life and pay special attention sustaining positive relationships. Make your mind firm and do come to a positive decision and not allow the worries to un-ease the power your mind and soul that can cause unhappiness in you.

We must free ourselves from fruitless worry.

Once a decision is carefully reached we should get busy carrying out our decisions and should not bother about all the anxieties that are about to come.

When we, or any of our colleagues or associates, are about to worry about a problem, we must write it out and think of the following questions: Instead of worrying about what people say, why not spend time trying to accomplish something they may admire. What if we just acted like everything was easy? How would your life be different if we stopped worrying about things we can't control and started focusing on the things we can? Let today be the day. We must free ourselves from fruitless worry, seize the day and take effective action on things we can change thus we would see that our lives changes for the betterment and we are on the right path of a sweet, good and happy living.

LEAVE WORRIES NOW
BE HAPPY ENJOY LIFE

CHAPTER 44

GET MORE SUCCESS AND HAPPINESS

If you are interested in getting more success and happiness within you, focus on all the ways as if you have already attained success. You need to focus on the thing and create a happy live within you. If you want love and affection, focus on all the people and the abundance of love that you have to give to them. If we want to have greater health, focus on all the ways that we are healthy, thus creating and delivering a good life within you. You need to admit that there are problems that you cannot change. But you can change the way of your thinking if you identify the main reason of the problem. And if you acknowledge the facts, that you have been negative or inactive in finding a solution to the problem, probably this will make it easier for you to become positive thus creating a new lease of life within you. It will make your life easier to lead a good and sweet life.

You must try to make goals

You must try to make goals. Making goals can give you a more positive outlook on life. People often tend to get bored with life and get the feeling that they are stuck to negative things which the result they often get the feeling of being depressed. Setting a direction for yourself and a goal would surely help you to move forward.

Mental attitude that can bring you peace and happiness

If you expecting to succeed, and are not afraid of failure, you have the best chance of staying positive and can create a very positive life within you. When you, or any of your associates, are tempted to worry about a problem, write out the solution and a definite answer to it. This helps a positive feeling to generate within you making you very positive to have a good living. Another thing you need to understand is that there are several ways to cultivate a mental attitude that can bring you peace and happiness and can carnage a good life within you. More of it if you fill your mind with thoughts of peace, courage, health, and hope, your life will be easy to live. You would get a happy feeling of life and mind if you let yourself to forget your own unhappiness, by trying to create a little happiness for others. You are best to yourself and to others.

The first step is to write down your worries

The first step is to write down your worries, which will help you make sense of them, and then decide on one small step you can take towards a solution. But to be very true no man in this world is free of obstacles or difficulties. Don't make worry your habit. Break this habit and stop all the negative and panic thoughts provoking your mind all the time. If you can't change the past, but you must not ruin the present by worrying about the future. Joy is what happens to us when we allow ourselves to recognize how good things really are. When we feel worried and depressed, we need to consciously form a smile on our faces and act upbeat until the happy feeling becomes genuine reality.

Happiness is what is needed most.

What makes to lead a happy life is not to get trapped into unnecessary unwanted worries and negative thoughts.

Don't create the feeling of depression and anger. Feelings of depression and hopelessness and or anger are even tougher to cope with on a consistent basis. When you are worried, you not only hurt yourself, but the limited support systems that are still holding on your mind but making you to get more and more worried and nothing is achieved in terms of success except the re-carnation of worries and worries thus leading you to be unhappy and worried all the time. Your actions breed confidence and courage. If you want to conquer fear, anger and worry do not sit ideal and just think about it. Let our deep worrying become advance thinking and planning. If you look into your own mind and heart, and you find nothing wrong there, what is there to worry about? Practically nothing what is there to fear about and again nothing? So why worry unnecessarily and make your present and future dark. Neglect all those which make your life unhappy.

Why being a negative person?

Why being a negative person and what do you get out of it being a depression dejected and sad man.? Why not turn your thoughts to be a positive person simply it is a question of tilting your mind towards a positive side of thing. See both the aspects of a situation and ways the pros and cons of both the sides and try to abolish the negativity in you. Be positive strong and you will remain happy for ever. We all have different roles that we play in the lives of people we love and care about. Our actions and how well we play our part has a direct influence on their life, so we better get in there and give our best performance. Tell them with how much you care in the capacity that you're in. At the end of the day, money is just a means to an end. Nothing more.

If you're grinding and struggling to make ends meet and buried under piles of debt, that's pretty stressful. Once you have your basic needs met though, more money only makes you happier up to a certain point. Money cannot buy you happiness. You need to generate it yourself. Someone will always be better than you at something, but it does not matter. Be inspired by them, using it to push yourself further, and nothing more. If they can do it, why cannot you?

Are you are interested in getting more happiness?.

If you are interested in getting more happiness focus on all the ways as if you have already attained success. You need to focus on the thing and create a live within you. If you want love and affection, focus on all the people and the abundance of love that you have to give to them.

Worrisome thoughts reproduce faster.

Worrisome thoughts reproduce faster so one of the most powerful ways to stop the spiral of worry is simply to disclose the worry to a friend. Practice happy gratitude daily. Take three minutes at the end of your day to chill and write down a small list of the things that can make you smile, laugh, or that you're glad are a part of your life. There's something to be grateful about, especially when you look down at that list and realize that a lot of people have it worse off than you do and could use a few of those things. Simply being an optimist will not solve all your problems, but what's the alternative is to keep your mind and heart cool and always have happy and positive feeling and think that life is to live happily. There isn't much sense in being anything else.

If you're constantly filling your head with negative thoughts, odds are they'll lead you straight towards negative actions, self-doubt and increase the general happiness of life isn't a cool place to live at all. Think of each setback as a challenge to see the positive, spin the situation back around, making it better than it was before and start living in a good and sweet manner.

What do we get out of unhappiness?

We may feel largely uncomfortable, when worries attack our thoughts and mind. While we are consuming more worries we are far too busy to do anything else to fix the real problem and would rather find it hard to get into a smart solution. Thus resulting in a fact that you spend your evenings worrying only without even bothering to find some time to know its cause We get nothing out of worrying except only to think and cry and become unhappy. We do not get anything out of unhappiness. Another thing is that we may feel largely uncomfortable, when worries attack our thoughts and mind which makes worrying about a situation an easier option to get depressed and diffused. While we are consuming more worries we are far too busy to do anything else to fix the real problem and would rather find it hard to get into a smart solution. Thus resulting in a fact that we spend our evenings worrying only without even bothering to find some time to search a sweet happiness within us. Negative thought which are provoking our mind, about the uncertainties and the negativities, as to what will happen tomorrow creates unnecessary worries and worries are repetitive thoughts associated with feelings of anxiety in anticipation of some negative future event which may end in a failure.

Negative thoughts create unnecessary worries

Whether the worries are about financial crisis, family problems, work, health or any topic of concern, the anxious feelings and negative thoughts produced are always distinctly unpleasant thus making us unhappy all the time. We get nothing being a negative and unhappy man. We must not forget that if we tend to worry they will never rob tomorrow of its sorrows, but will only deny today of its meaning happiness and joys. Negative thoughts only produce worries and worrying is actually a form of superstition and creates false images in our mind and that is the main reason and cause which makes and leads us to this point of imagination. A human being can survive almost anything, as long as he or she sees the end in sight, starts analyzing his positive thoughts and starts analyzing his unhappiness.

We need to fore see the coming trouble first.

We must not forgot that if something bad or good is to happen it is sure to happen, whether we worry or not. Let us put our energy into today and stop worrying about the future and past. We should not foresee trouble, or worry about what may never happen as past is dead and gone forever and future is uncertain and yet to come. Positive thinking our brave attitude and our courage will ward off everything and bring happiness in our lives. The basic facts we should know about worry. The basic techniques to analyze worry and how to break the worry habit before it breaks us. These are the simple ways where we can concentrate and get rid of worries prevailing in our thoughts, remove all the negativity in our live and start living a positive good and happy life.

Think of good and positive ways of Happy Living.

Annalise positive ways of happy living and get to see the reasons and facts of worry. To avoid reoccurrence of worries, concentrate on prayers as prayers are the best source of remedies of the prevailing worries. Think good ways of living and starting praying. The more you pray, the less you'll panic. The more you worship, the less you worry. There is nothing that wastes the body like worry, and anyone who has any faith in God should need not to worry about anything whatsoever is to happen in future. Positive thinking is the creation of good imagination and good imagination is the creation of sweet and happy living.

Happiness comes with Positive living and sweet thoughts

If you know that the circumstance is beyond your control or power change than revise it to your liking. Just try to put a stop-less order on your worries. Don't permit little things which become insects of life to ruin your happiness. Co-operate with the inevitable. Decide just how much anxiety a thing may be worth and refuse to give in anymore.

All the happiness is not given in one go it comes slowly and slowly with positive thinking.

Have worry under your control. If your worries center around, pay special attention to remain positive and be happy. Keep yourself happy, treat your worried thoughts as valuable signals. How to keep from worrying about criticism? Simply unjust criticism and think positively and do often discard a bad compliment. It often means that you have aroused jealousy and envy. Let's keep a record of the fool things we have done and stop criticizing ourselves.

Cause of unhappiness is Negative way of living life

The utmost cause of worry is our negative thinking as it leads us to the state of depression. Living will change for the better-If You Think Positive. Our negative thinking and attitude towards suffering and depression becomes very important because it can affect how we cope with suffering when it arises. Depression is nourished by a lifetime of un-grieved and unforgiven causes. Times will change for the better when you change. Worry is a misuse of the imagination. Worry is most often a prideful way of thinking that you have more control over life and its circumstances than you actually do. Positive Thinking leads your way to good and happiness. An art of Good and Happy Living.

Neglect worries keep yourself happy.

Neglect worries keep yourself happy, treat your worried thoughts as valuable signals. These are the fundamental facts you should be familiar about worries. A huge factor to stay happy is to cater your worries around, an important relationship in your life and pay special attention sustaining positive relationships. Worries are there to motivate information gathering and problem-solving. Make your mind firm and do come to a positive decision as come what we will not allow the worries to entire our mind and soul.

What if we just acted like everything was easy?

Once a decision is carefully reached we should get busy carrying out our decisions and should not bother about all the anxieties that are about to come. When we, or any of our colleagues or associates, are about to worry about a problem, we must write it out and think positively of the questions.

Instead of worrying about what people say of you, why not spend time trying to accomplish something they will admire. What if we just acted like everything was easy? How would your life be different if you stopped worrying about things we can't control and started focusing on the things we can? Let today be the day. Free yourself from fruitless worry, seize the day and take effective action on things you can change. We would change ourselves for the betterment if we start thinking in positive terms. Positive thinking is what is required of us and simply worrying about the future things or as to what will happen in the next moment will certainly deprive us of good and happy living that we are about gather or get in the next hour.

Another cause of getting worried or unhappy is the attachment

Attachment brings worry. If you have a problem and you come up with the answer, you stop worrying immediately.

Our minds can be dishonest, persuading us that we are worrying about something, when our deepest fear is entirely different. No-one likes to admit that they've chosen to worry. The first step is to write down your worries, which will help you make sense of them, and then decide on one small step you can take towards a solution. But to be very true no man in this world is free of obstacles or difficulties.

Don't make worry your habit. Break this habit and stop all the negative and panic thoughts provoking your mind all the time if you want to remain a happy person and lead a happy good and sweet life. Feelings of depression and angry are even tougher to cope with on a consistent basis.

When you are worried, you not only hurt yourself, but the limited support systems that are still holding on your mind making you to get more and more worried and nothing is achieved in terms of success except the re-carnation of worries and worries Joy is what happens to us when we allow ourselves to recognize how good things really are.

Practically nothing what is there to fear about?

So why worry unnecessarily and make your present and future dark. Why being a negative person and what do you get out of it being a depression dejected and sad man.? Why not turn your thoughts to be a positive person simply it is a question of tilting your mind towards a positive side of thing. See both the aspects of a situation and ways the pros and cons of both the sides and try to abolish the negativity in you. You will surely be a happy man.

Think of the best the best is sure to happen

Think of the best the best is sure to happen and if you think of the worst the worst will come. Better come forward wake up and think positive first. Positive persons always succeed in life whatever be the circumstances and the negative often dig a death trap for themselves. So why be a negative person why you have all the qualities of being a positive man. Surround yourself with friends and people that are better than you in areas that you want to improve in.

LEAVE WORRIES NOW
BE HAPPY ENJOY LIFE

CHAPTER 45

HAPPINESS IS NECCESSARY

For An Art of Happy Living

Remember three aspects - naturalness, simplicity and belongingness. Just open up your heart and be natural. Next is living a simple life. Living with the confidence will get whatever is needed, that is simplicity. Right or wrong, we are what we are. We need to tone our life accordingly and if we live like this naturally, then there will not be any fear. There will be no doubts or blocks in life. This is the important mantra of Art of Sweet Living. Another important thing is that if we cannot get some good sunshine, we can always lighten up our thoughts with brighter lights of happy living. We can have ample of lunch of positive thinking. To avoid negative thoughts we need to take frequent walks. No man is indispensable and no man is not capable of positive thinking. Let us make ourselves happy and life become a sweet living.

Happiness is a state of mind.

We know the saying, that "Happiness is a state of mind". And state of mind is what we think and what we do or act in a peaceful manner without being getting worried or depressed. If you are interested in getting more happiness, to get it through positive thinking. All we need to do is to focus on all the directions on positive thinking and happy living as if we have already attained success.

We need to focus on the thing and create a life within us. If we want love and affection, entertain people and give them the abundance of love. If we want to have greater health, pay attention on all the ways that make us healthy, thus creating and delivering a good life within us by thinking in positive ways. We need to understand and admit that there are problems that we cannot change. But we can change the ways of our thinking and if we identify the main reason of the problem we can remove all the obstacles coming in our way of leading a sweet and happy life. And if we acknowledge the fact, that we have been negative or inactive in finding a solution to the problem, this will make it easier for us to become positive thus creating a new lease of life within us.

Positive thinking will surely make us happy.

Another thing to understand is that we must try to make our goals. Making goals can give us a more positive outlook on life. People often tend to get bored with life and get the feeling that they are stuck to negative things with the result they often get the feeling of being depressed dejected and monotonous and become unhappy in life. Setting a direction and a goal for ourselves, would surely help us to move forward. If we are expecting to succeed, and are not afraid of failure, we stand the best chance of staying positive and thus can create a very positive life within us.

Mental attitude that can bring you peace and happiness.

Another thing you need to understand is that there are several ways to cultivate a mental attitude that can bring you peace and happiness and can carnage a good life within you.

More of it if you fill your mind with thoughts of peace, courage, health, and hope, your life will be easy to live. If you think in positive terms you would get a happy feeling of life and mind you if you let yourself to forget your own unhappiness, by trying to create a little happiness for others you are sure to get happiness in your live. You are best to yourself. The perfect way to conquer worry is the Prayer of God. You should do things in the order of their importance.

Learn to think in positive terms.

When you face a problem, solve it then and there, by thinking positively and if you have the facts of making a decision, make a decision fast and do not linger on. Learn to think in positive terms organize the things, deputise, and supervise straight away by coming to decision. To keep yourself from worrying about criticism, do not even try to get mixed with your enemies, because if you do you will hurt yourself far more than we hurting them. You will fall prey to negative thinking and this in turn will lead you unhappiness in life. Simply postponing it would spoil your good thoughts and there is every likelihood your mind may get into negative activities and start thinking in negative manner. Therefore think positive, write down a list of things that make you positive, however big, small, likely or unlikely. Then work to make them occur more often. Look for moments of joy and savor them. Recognise your good happening every day. Be positive think positive and be happy.

Happiness is your own choice and decision

You may also feel that life has become terrible for you to live and you are carrying no hope that someone would be there to rescue you.

Happiness is your own choice and decision. Each of us can be as happy as we make up our minds to be. We can, if we want, fill up our days with positive attitude chatter and laughter. To be happy, we need to concentrate only on happy thoughts. Our friends are always there to give us some moral support. Spending time and engaging ourselves in worthwhile positive activities could give us a very enjoyable and satisfying feeling. Nothing feels better than having group support and talking in terms of positive thinking. Good friends are quite important and their company generally lightened up our spirits. This makes us to think in positive manner and to get to know such friends we simply have to be friendly with ourselves, and then the friendships will naturally follow us and make our lives happy.

Only way to find happiness is not to expect gratitude.

Let us remember that the only way to find happiness is not to expect gratitude, but to give for the joy of giving. Let us build a happy life within us generate peace and a healthy atmosphere around us. This will help us to lead a peaceful happy and prosperous life and we would find ourselves to be happier than before. We need to understand the power of positive thinking and its support and we have not to underestimate it strength and support. Don't we feel so good when someone pats us on our back and gives us some words of encouragement during your most challenging times and difficult times and advises us to remain positive and think positive just hug or embrace someone with positive attitude someday? We will see that we have almost changed our life. The ghosts of the past have to be exorcised. We may be working in any field, the key to success is our outlook.

Sometimes we may think that no road is left for us from where we can achieve the happiness of life. One need not to forgot that we need to eat well do plenty of exercise and do not skip meals It is a known fact that physical exercise is known to stimulate our veins and get to strengthen our minds that lift depression and anxiety, so we need to walk, swim, run or whatever we like doing best above all we must move ahead in direction where our mind can generate electricity to think in positive directly and bring immense happiness to us.

Difficulties and storms may come and go.

In our lives difficulties and storms may come and go in the form of reversals, but if we have the power of positive thinking and foundation of inner fulfillment we would be able to deal with it with a very clear practical mind and with this positive thinking these storms will not kill us nor will disrupt us. There could be numberless reasons for which we keep on worrying. We may be worried about our health, wealth, loved ones, friends, the happening of yesterday and the follow happenings of tomorrow, the environment or the world politics, but these can be dealt with firm mind and fearless worry if we generate within ourselves the power of positive thinking within ourselves and try to be happy all the time.

The best thing about happiness is that we get it is free.

We don't have to pay or we do not have to open any account to be happy. We don't have to pay monthly rent for it either. WE just have to change our perspective, our views on what we are seeing and feeling. Happiness is not something which is quite readymade. It comes from our own actions and deeds.

Angriness and happiness don't mix.

We must dig out the angriness in us, and see that the happiness has shown and seeded a place to grow its roots. The ultimate goal of life should be to get happiness and not get involved into unnecessary worries falling in the death trap of defeats and failures. The essence of life is not in the great victories and grand failures, but in the simple joys. The purpose of our lives is to be happy.

If you want to be happy, be positive first practice meditation.

Laugh when you can, apologize when you should, and let go of what you can't change.

Think positive and just visualize that what is stored in destiny would not be negative. If you want to be happy, be positive first practice meditation. If you want, others to be happy practice compassion. Whoever is happy will make others happy, too.

Happiness doesn't depend on any superficial conditions.

Let us be very sure and let us keep in mind that happiness doesn't depend on any superficial conditions, it is governed by our mental attitude only. Our greatest gift to others is to be happy and to radiate our happiness to the entire world. Happiness is a guide to direction, not a place to hide. As a happy person, we radiate happiness to the world. We need to visualise our light radiating throughout the world, passing from person to person until it encircles the globe. Resolve to keep happy, and you shall form an invincible host against difficulties.

The path to happiness is forgiveness.

The positive persons often dance to the happy tunes of their lives. The path to happiness is forgiveness of everyone and gratitude for everything. Happiness fills our heart each day and our whole life through with clean thoughts. Any day would be a wonderful day if we do not to take life so seriously. Happiness is not about being a winner it is about being gentle with life being gentle within us. Happiness blooms in the presence of self-respect and the absence of ego. Love yourself. Love everyone around you. Love everyone in the whole world. When you're feeling depressed or anxious, close your eyes and try to visualize a guided positive imaginary thing. First breathe deeply and relax. How important it is to consistently reach for positive, uplifting, inspirational thoughts. Thought that promote aliveness and abundance. Thoughts that make you feel good. Imagine that you are already a positive person and you love life.

Happiness can only be achieved if you have a positive mind.

The only thing between us and our desire, to be happy, is one single fact: we are not happy because we often fall into the death trap of depression and wholly because of our negative thoughts. Absence of positive thinking, has eluded us of our great happiness and left us far behind. This very little known fact has kept many of us from reaching our goal of happiness.

Throw away all your negative thoughts and worries, concentrate on the goals to be achieved, on the ray of happiness in you and make sure that you are not falling again into the path of negativity.

Happiness is a state of mind only and not the thoughts of negatives, and it quite true that happiness can only be achieved if you have a positive mind and a clear attitude of being a positive person. Happiness and positivity go hand in hand. If you are positive you are a happy person and if you possess negativity you would land yourself to be a very negative person thus ruining your life for what of nothing with the result you become an unhappy person and you remain aloof from leading a sweet good and happy living.

LEAVE WORRIES NOW
BE HAPPY ENJOY LIFE

CHAPTER 46

DISCARD BAD LIVINGAND START HAPPY LIVING

Happiness is our own choice and decision. Each of us can be as happy as we make up our minds to be. We can, if we want, fill up our days with positive attitude chatter and laughter. To be happy, we need to concentrate only on happy thoughts. The ghosts of the past have to be exorcised. We may be working in any field, the key to success is our outlook. Sometimes we may think that no road is left for us from where you can achieve the happiness of life. There may be chances that someone who was there with us before might hold on to us when we are on the dark side of the life.

Positive thinking and happy living is state of mind.

Positive thinking and happy living is state of mind and happiness is something we cannot earn or buy. We need to remember that people and things alone, won't make us happy. Our own efforts not to get worried or depressed make us happy. Positive living make us happy. We ought to remember the saying, that "Positive living along can bring happiness as it is a state of mind".

The ultimate goal of life should be to get happiness.

The ultimate goal of life should be to get happiness and not get involved into unnecessary worries falling in the death trap of defeats and failures.

The essence of life is not in the great victories and grand failures, but in the simple joys. The purpose of our lives is to be happy. Laugh when we can, apologize when we should, and let go of what we can't change. Let us think positive and just visualize that what is stored in destiny would not be negative. If we want to be happy, practice meditation. If we want, others to be happy practice compassion. Whoever is happy will make others happy, too. Thus we can lead our path to happy sweet and good living.

Our greatest gift to others is to be happy.

Let us be very sure and let us keep in mind that happiness doesn't depend on any superficial conditions, it is governed by our mental attitude only. Our greatest gift to others is to be happy and to radiate our happiness to the entire world. Happiness is a guide to direction, not a place to hide. As a happy person, we radiate happiness to the world. We need to visualize our light radiating throughout the world, passing from person to person until it encircles the globe. Resolve to keep happy, and your joy and you shall form an invincible host against difficulties.

The positive persons often dance to the happy tunes.

The positive persons often dance to the happy tunes of their lives. The path to happiness is forgiveness of everyone and gratitude for everything. Happiness fills your heart each day and your whole life through with clean thoughts. Any day would be a wonderful day if you do not to take life so seriously. Happiness is not about being a winner it is about being gentle with life being gentle within you.

Happiness blooms in the presence of self-respect and the absence of ego. Love yourself. Love everyone around you. Love everyone in the whole world.

Happiness is not about being a winner it is about being gentle

When you're feeling depressed or anxious, close your eyes and try to visualize a guided positive imaginary thing. First breathe deeply and relax. How important it is to consistently reach for positive, uplifting, inspirational thoughts. Thought that promote aliveness and abundance. Thoughts that make you feel good. Happiness is not about being a winner it is about being gentle. The only thing between us and our desire, to be happy, is one single fact: we are not happy because we often fall into the death trap of depression and wholly because of our negative thoughts.

Throw away all your negative thoughts.

Throw away all your negative thoughts and worries, concentrate on the goals to be achieved, on the ray of happiness in you and make sure that you are not falling again into the path of negativity. Positive and happy living is not state of mind only it is the discernment of the negatives thoughts .Be a positive thinker and ignore reality in favor of aspirational thoughts. It is more about taking a proactive approach to life. Instead of feeling hopeless or overwhelmed, positive thinking and happy living allows to tackle life's challenges by looking for effective ways to resolve conflict and come up with creative solutions to problems. It might not be easy, but the positive person will surely win and lead a sweet happy and good life.

Happiness in life comes through the doors of positive thoughts;

We do not even realize which one is left open. We have so many reasons to cry and at the same time plenty of reasons to smile as well. Keeping our dreams and hope alive might be a reason that success and happiness will come our way again. We ought to know that happiness alone does not stand for anything, but it is on our way of thinking that how do we keep ourselves happy in life. Ending up our lives does not lead us to our destination but of course proves we are supposed to be cowards who know not to unfold the doors of belief in God and in ourselves.

Failure and disappointment are part of our life.

Failure and disappointment are part of our life. The only thing is that we need to face them boldly and courageously and try our best to solve the problem. We must not forget to believe in God whatever our situation may be we need to make our faith strong enough not be let down, rather we would break the knees of sorrows and force it to die and lead happy lives. We should not surrender but must find out ways to come out of our worries, anxieties and difficulties.

Happy living is sure to make our life a good and sweet one.

We ought not to indulge ourselves into the darkness of the room but find out the doors to free ourselves from unnecessary fear and worries. We must belief in ourselves and our hearts, and believe in the ones who love us and not the ones whom we love. We must not fall on the negative side of a thing. The experience has taught us that we should buy some strength, hope and positive ness from our loved ones to help ourselves in such a situation rather than surrendering our lives to God as it is a precious gift of God which is equipped with full of joy and happiness we need to help ourselves in these critical moments and live with considerable optimism. Happy living is sure to make our life good and sweet.

We should always try to be positive and happy

It is the real time when you keep on revealing the truth of our lives and relations, do not fall on the reverse side but think how good it was that because of the hard times of our lives we could well judge about them. We should always try to be positive and should think that whatever is happening, it is the positive side or consequence of that incident in would be on the positive side of our imagination. With all these thoughts, I would request my readers to implement some good thoughts in their life. That would make things easier to be tackled by them. We should accept the situation and fight it with more determination.

In this world nothing is good or bad and only thinking makes it so.

We ought to know that advice from people around us will help us to overcome from the any drastic situation. Also we have to always minimize the stress as it gives nothing but takes away joy and happiness from our lives. And finally we need to take things casually and fight with it seriously. A clear minded person looks for good qualities in the other person, whereas a negative mind always looks for the fault in the other person and also a negative mind always looks for the fault. An optimist goes forward keeping in mind the past, a pessimist thinks of the future and reverts back to the past. In fact negative thoughts are our greatest enemies.

Experience the happiness in all circumstances by maintaining better relationships.

Sadness cannot touch a person with a positive attitude. It increases the decision of making power. Creative way of thoughts appears in the mind. Positive thoughts of happy living teach us the art of finding solutions to any problem. Optimism is something what we do. Anxiety and other negative emotions are known to be detrimental to the body, especially to our immune systems, and having an optimistic nature seems to protect against those effects. People who are supposed to be optimistic, about their future, are sure to lead a sweet good and happy life. Their secret of happiness is that they do exercise, do not indulge in in smoking and often follow a good and better diet. Whenever we are unhappy, if we analyze the reason for our unhappiness, it is because life is not matching our expectations. We need to experience the happiness in all circumstances by maintaining better understanding and relationships with all.

LEAVE WORRIES NOW
BE HAPPY ENJOY LIFE

CHAPTER 47

STOP WORRING -START LIVING

At time we may think that there is no road is left for us from where we can achieve the happiness of our lives. We may also feel that life has become terrible for us to live and we are carrying new hope that someone would come to rescue us. There may be chances that someone who was there with us before might have held on to us when we were on the dark side of the life.

It is important for us to stay open to laughter and humor.

Even when we are facing challenges, it is important for us to stay open to laughter and humor. Sometimes, simply recognizing the potential humor in a situation can lessen our stress and brighten our outlook. Seeking out sources of humor such as watching a funny sitcom or reading jokes online can help us to think more positively. The experience has taught us that we should buy some strength, hope and positive ness from our loved ones to help ourselves in such a situation rather than surrendering as life is a precious gift of God and is equipped with full of joy and happiness if we help ourselves in these critical moments and live with considerable optimism. Happiness in life comes through the doors of positive thoughts; we do not even realize which one is left open.

We have so many reasons to cry and at the same time plenty of reasons to smile as well.

Keeping our dreams and hope alive might be a reason that success and happiness will come our way again. We ought to know that happiness alone does not stand for anything, but it is on our way of thinking that how do we keep ourselves happy in life. Ending up our lives does not lead us to our destination but of course proves we are supposed to be cowards who know not to unfold the doors of belief in God and in ourselves. But if our faith is strong enough we will not be let down, rather we would break the knees of sorrows and force it to die and lead happy lives.

We must find out ways to come out of our worries, anxieties and difficulties.

We should not surrender but must find out ways to come out of our worries, anxieties and difficulties. We ought not to indulge ourselves into the darkness of the room but find out the doors to free ourselves from unnecessary fear and worries. We must belief in ourselves and our hearts, and believe in the ones who love us and not the ones whom we love. We must not fall on the negative side of a thing. It is the real time when we keep on revealing the truth of our lives and relations. We should always try to be happy and should think that whatever is happening, it is the positive side. We should accept the situation and fight it with more determination. We must find out ways to come out of our worries, anxieties and difficulties in order for us to lead a happy sweet and good life.

Negative thoughts are our greatest enemies.

We ought to know that advice from people around us will help us to overcome from the any drastic situation.

Also we have to always minimize the stress as it gives nothing but takes away joy and happiness from our lives.

And finally we need to take things casually and fight with it seriously. A clear minded person looks for good qualities in the other person, whereas a negative mind always looks for the fault in the other person, whereas a negative mind always looks for the fault. An optimist goes forward keeping in mind the past, a pessimist thinks of the future and reverts back to the past. In fact negative thoughts are our greatest enemies. Experience the happiness in all circumstances by maintaining better relationships.

We need to analyise the reason for our unhappiness.

Whenever we are unhappy, if we analyze the reason for our unhappiness, it is because life is not matching our desires and expectations. We need to know and realize that nobody is perfect or flawless. If we try to change the way we look, talk and behave just to please others, and show our pride we will gradually become such a person that we ourselves won't recognize each other and would start and create unnecessary worries within us and our surrounding without being positive and will not start to live happily. We ought to stop worrying over unnecessary things be positive and live without fear. Living happily is the master key to all problems and worries. Forgot worries discard all problems take them lightly and behave as nothing serious has happened. This way we are sure to overcome all problems and lead a happy life. We need to understand that what people think of us is their concern, and not ours. If they think about us to be, too reticent or proud, it's really not our business. If every time we happen to meet some new fellows, we may wonder and imagine as what they think of us, and with this feeling in us we will never be able to live a trouble-free and hassle free life.

We are bound to fall into the trap of unnecessary worries denying us the startup of new and the happy living life.

Positive attitude is a quality of happy living.

We must think rationally. Is it in our hands or can we control what others think about us? Simply we need to ignore them, if we cannot, and live our lives the way we want to and find the ways to leave worries aside and start living a happy life. Let us make our way to happy living. It is a well-known fact that attitude decides how a natives or persons copes up with the day to day events of life. Attitude is the main influence a person's reaction to a situation in life. It sets the emotional undertone for a person to his likes or dislikes a situation even before he is acquainted with it. Positive attitude is a quality of happy living which is second to none in a human being. We acknowledge our children to say a big thank you from the time to time irrespective they being very little, we teach them to be grateful for everything that they receive. We attach so much importance to this attitude of gratitude that when our children fail to thank someone, we insist that they do it. That is what is needed to be avoided from time to time. We expect this in return from others when we help them or give them a gift. We call a person discourteous and rude when they do not say thank us in return. Though we attach so much importance to this attitude, as we grow into teenage and adult years we find ourselves becoming ungrateful or taking things for granted. We lose touch with the very same qualities that we instill in our children. We take for granted our life, our health, our families, the people in our lives, the things that our loved ones do for us to make our lives easier and things that we possess.

The attitude of positive or happy living speaks a lot about a person.

It denotes about changing negative attitudes and making positive thinking a positive a good habit. Thinking positively and a positive attitude help us to appreciate and value ourselves, our potential and all that we have. It ensures that we do not take our abilities for granted. It makes us look at ourselves as special people with a special set of abilities and potential. It banishes the feelings of inadequacy and insecurity that arises from unfair comparisons with others. It helps us to appreciate people for who they are and not magnify what they are not and their little flaws. It drives away prejudice and makes us approach life with an open mind. It predisposes us to react to the daily events of life in a positive manner and help us to look at the brighter side of life. Make us optimistic. It gives hope and helps us look forward to life with anticipation making our lives happier and happier day by day. We need to know that positive thinking takes the focus away from what we don't have, to appreciating and making good use of what we have. It is closely connected to our emotional wellbeing and happiness. We feel loved and at peace with ourselves for a major part of our lives when we make this attitude ours. This adds and helps us to get rid of greed, amenity, bitterness, jealousy, and promotes a healthy and nurturing attitude towards others, which in turn gets reciprocated and we feel the sense of healthy living. On the face of it we ought to know that a positive and good living is an attitude that makes you feel good about who you are, what you do, and what your potentials are. This attitude impels you to utilize all that you are endowed with as a person, to achieve the highest possible goals.

When we have this attitude, we are able to work without any external pressure to perform but there is sufficient pressure and motivation from within.

Positive thinking and a positive attitude of happy life is a joy for ever

The possessing of happy living is like any other habit, so we need to follow the routine of habit formation here as well. You will win new friends and admirers without having to impress them or conform to the pressure of doing things their way. You will be bubbling with life. You will be rearing to go and accomplish all you can with your new found confidence. The best part of adopting the 'positive thinking and a positive attitude of gratitude is that, you will be able to enjoy the smallest pleasures of nature with a heightened sense of satisfaction and awe. We can see and watch a beautiful flower and carry that joy in our mind for future enjoyment with a clear positive habit. We can go back to work freshen and can use it as an object to meditate on when we feel stressed. When we have this attitude, we are able to work without any external pressure to perform but there is sufficient pressure and motivation from within. The habit of happy living is like any other habit, so we need to follow the routine of habit formation here as well.

**LEAVE WORRIES NOW
BE HAPPY ENJOY LIFE**

CHAPTER 48

BRING BACK YOUR HAPPY DAYS

We need to remember that as we possibly as we can we should make it a point to eat a more balanced, and healthy diet even though we may very little money left with us. We have intake of lot of greens vegetables and with variety of fruit and nuts which are all super healthy food for us, and which are less expensive than meats, cheeses, and processed foods! Their nitrifying value will energize and elevate our body, and knowing this that we are treating ourselves will surely refresh our minds. If we look for rich food rich in vitamins and other useful ingredients which include nuts, soya beans and fatty fish we would get more nutrition value. We must cut back on the caffeine drinks, alcohol. We don't have to quit, but reducing the intake of them will help reduce anxiety and stress from time to time. Exercise is one of health sport that our body needs most. It may be yoga, cross training, or even a simple walking in the park. This helps keeping our body active and will also help to grow our outlook. If we make it hobby we would enjoy the most. Whether its art, photography, music focusing on something other than the worry factor it will give our mind some good atmosphere to breathe off and would generate a good behavior within us. The other refreshing factor is naturally our sleep. We need not be reminded of this. Our body is probably begging us for it when we are in the middle of hard times. We may be drawn to maintain good sleeping habits. Maintain a consistent sleep schedule, but allow yourself some leeway. If we sleep peacefully let our body get about 8 hours of sleep we get the best results.

If you're just starting to have those thoughts, speak to your physician or your therapist. They may prescribe something to help steer you back to the center, emotionally. It may be the act of talking about it is therapeutic enough, but don't assume that. Leave that call to the professionals. Having goals which are set again and again after each one is achieved will give you a mindset or target to strive for which leads to success, with success becomes natural positive attitude. With all costiveness, goals and success builds a higher potential and belief within yourself. Setting realistic goals that you know you can achieve by staying positive is a great beginning to success. Your attitude around your friends, family and public people really tells them who you are, being positive instead of negative makes an excellent first impression on anybody. Positive means to be absolute, clear-cut, definite, forward-looking and expressively firm with a decision. Having a positive attitude toward something means you are willing to commit and do the work without complaint, which leads to goals. You realize that what appears negative today will change tomorrow. Nothing stays the same. Whether you are positive or negative, the situation does not change. So, we mind as well be positive. As with any habit, the habit of remaining positive in all situations takes practice and a commitment to yourself to take control. But start small, start paying attention to your emotions, start by wanting to change. Don't hold onto anything that bothers your mind. It can only hurt your health and it won't help your problems at all. The people that live the longest in this world do not hold grudges or hold onto negative feelings. Visualize your worries on a large chalkboard in your mind. Watch yourself take a big eraser and erase the problems. Every time the thoughts come back into your head, see yourself with the eraser again. Therefore do not worry about tomorrow, for tomorrow will worry about itself. Each day has enough trouble of its own.

Do not anticipate trouble, or worry about what may never happen. Keep in the sunlight. Imagine every day to be the last of a life surrounded with hopes, cares, anger and fear. The hours that come unexpectedly will be much the more grateful. The mind that is anxious about future events is miserable. Present fears are less than horrible imaginings. Let us be of good cheer, remembering that the misfortunes hardest to bear are those that never happen, focus on the positive aspects of their lives, rather than on the negative setbacks. "Feeling confident affects the way we perceive our situations and how we decide to manage them. Don't waste your life in doubts and fears: spend yourself on the work before you, well assured that the right performance of this hour's duties will be the best preparation for the hours or ages that follow it. It is not work that kills men, it is worry. Work is healthy; you can hardly put more on a man than he can bear. But worry is rust upon the blade. It is not movement that destroys the machinery, but friction. Never let life's hardships disturb you ... no one can avoid problems, not even saints or sages. As with any habit, the habit of remaining positive in all situations takes practice and a commitment to yourself to take control. Life is what you make it, so make it a happy one!! Don't worry on things that may not happen, life is to short to worry to much. Smile and be happy

LEAVE WORRIES NOW
BE HAPPY ENJOY LIFE

CHAPTER 49

OUR OTHER PUBLICATION

ARE ON SALE

"MICROSCOPY OF ASTROLOGY"

"MICROSCOPY OF NUMEROLOGY"

"MICROSCOPY OF REMEDIES"

MICROSCOPY OF HAPPY LIVING

MICROSCOPY OF TRANSITING PLANETS

LEAVE WORRIES NOW
BE HAPPY ENJOY LIFE

CHAPTER 50

OUR CONTACT ADDRESS:

PLEASE SEND YOUR QUERIES TO:

BALDEV BHATIA

CONSULTANT-NUMEROLOGY-ASTROLOGY

C-63, FIRST FLOOR

MALVIYA NAGAR

NEW DELHI-110017

INDIA

TEL NO 919810075249

TEL NO 91 11 26686856

TEL NO 91 7503280786

TEL NO 91 7702735880

LEAVE WORRIES NOW
BE HAPPY ENJOY LIFE
CHAPTER 51

OUR MOST SOUGHT WEB SITES:

HTTP://WWW.ASTROLOGYBB.COM

HTTP://WWW.BBASTROLOGY.COM

HTTP://WWW.BALDEVBHATIA.COM

HTTP://WWW.BALDEVBHATIA.US

HTTP://WWW.BALDEVBHATIA.ORG

HTTP://WWW.BALDEVBHATIA.INFO

HTTP://WWW.BALDEVBHATIA.NET

HTTP://WWW.BALDEVBHATIA.BIZ

HTTP://WWW.BALDEVBHATIA.IN

LEAVE WORRIES NOW
BE HAPPY ENJOY LIFE

CHAPTER 52

SPECIAL NOTE

FROM THE AUTHOR BALDEV BHATIA

THANK YOU FOR READING MY BOOK

MY SINCERE PRAYERS

FOR ALL MY READERS

"GOD BLESS YOU ALL"

"ANY ONE WHO READS AND KEEPS THIS BOOK AS HOLY MANUSCRIPT, GOD IS SURE TO BLESS HIM, WITH ALL THE PEACE, HAPPINESS, WEALTH, HEALTH AND PROSPERITY OF THIS UNIVERSE"

BALDEV BHATIA

www.ingramcontent.com/pod-product-compliance
Lightning Source LLC
Chambersburg PA
CBHW060234290526
45789CB00001B/48